Evidence-Based Dentistry

Editor

ROBERT J. WEYANT

DENTAL CLINICS OF NORTH AMERICA

www.dental.theclinics.com

January 2019 • Volume 63 • Number 1

ELSEVIER

1600 John F. Kennedy Boulevard • Suite 1800 • Philadelphia, Pennsylvania, 19103-2899

http://www.dental.theclinics.com

DENTAL CLINICS OF NORTH AMERICA Volume 63, Number 1
January 2019 ISSN 0011-8532, ISBN: 978-0-323-65496-8

Editor: John Vassallo; j.vassallo@elsevier.com
Developmental Editor: Laura Fisher

Dental Clinics of North America (ISSN 0011-8532) is published quarterly by Elsevier Inc., 360 Park Avenue South, New York, NY 10010-1710. Months of issue are January, April, July, and October. Business and Editorial Offices: 1600 John F. Kennedy Boulevard, Suite 1800, Philadelphia, PA 19103-2899. Periodicals postage paid at New York, NY and additional mailing offices. Subscription prices are $304.00 per year (domestic individuals), $603.00 per year (domestic institutions), $100.00 per year (domestic students/residents), $366.00 per year (Canadian individuals), $782.00 per year (Canadian institutions), $424.00 per year (international individuals), $782.00 per year (international institutions), and $200.00 per year (international and Canadian students/residents). International air speed delivery is included in all *Clinics* subscription prices. All prices are subject to change without notice. **POSTMASTER:** Send address changes to *Dental Clinics of North America*, Elsevier Health Sciences Division, Subscription Customer Service, 3251 Riverport Lane, Maryland Heights, MO 63043. **Customer Service (orders, claims, online, change of address): Elsevier Health Sciences Division, Subscription Customer Service, 3251 Riverport Lane, Maryland Heights, MO 63043. Tel: 1-800-654-2452 (U.S. and Canada). Fax: 314-447-8029. E-mail: journalscustomer service-usa@elsevier.com (for print support); journalsonlinesupport-usa@elsevier.com (for online support).**

Reprints. For copies of 100 or more, of articles in this publication, please contact the Commercial Reprints Department, Elsevier Inc., 360 Park Avenue South, New York, NY 10010-1710. Tel.: 212-633-3874; Fax: 212-633-3820; E-mail: reprints@elsevier.com.

The Dental Clinics of North America is covered in *MEDLINE/PubMed (Index Medicus), Current Contents/Clinical Medicine, ISI/BIOMED* and *Clinahl.*

Contributors

EDITOR

ROBERT J. WEYANT, MS, DMD, DrPH
Professor and Chair, Department of Dental Public Health, University of Pittsburgh School of Dental Medicine, Pittsburgh, Pennsylvania, USA

AUTHORS

SARAH R. BAKER, BSc, PhD, AFBPsS
Professor of Psychology as applied to Dentistry, The School of Clinical Dentistry, University of Sheffield, Sheffield, United Kingdom

BEN BALEVI, DDS, MSc
Private Practice, Associate Professor, Faculty of Medicine, University of British Columbia, Vancouver, British Columbia, Canada

PAUL R. BROCKLEHURST, BDS, BSc (Hons), MDPH, PhD, FFGDP, FDS RCS (Eng)
Professor of Health Services Research, Normal Site, Bangor University, Bangor, United Kingdom

DONALD L. CHI, DDS, PhD
Associate Professor, Department of Oral Health Sciences, University of Washington, School of Dentistry, Seattle, Washington, USA

YASMI O. CRYSTAL, DMD, MSc, FAAPD
Clinical Professor, Pediatric Dentistry, New York University College of Dentistry, New York, New York, USA

MARGHERITA FONTANA, DDS, PhD
Department of Cariology, Restorative Sciences and Endodontics, Clifford Nelson Endowed Professor of Dentistry, University of Michigan School of Dentistry, Ann Arbor, Michigan, USA

KATHERINE FRANCE, DMD, MBE
Assistant Professor of Oral Medicine, University of Pennsylvania School of Dental Medicine, Philadelphia, Pennsylvania, USA

JULIE FRANTSVE-HAWLEY, PhD
Department of Guidelines and Publishing, American College of Chest Physicians, Glenview, Illinois, USA

JANE GILLETTE, DDS, MPH
Director, Sprout Oral Health, Bozeman, Montana, USA

CARLOS GONZALEZ-CABEZAS, DDS, MSD, PhD
Department of Cariology, Restorative Sciences and Endodontics, Richard Christensen Collegiate Professor of Oral and Craniofacial Global Initiatives, University of Michigan School of Dentistry, Ann Arbor, Michigan, USA

ELLIOT V. HERSH, DMD, MS, PhD
Professor, Department of Oral Surgery and Pharmacology, University of Pennsylvania School of Dental Medicine, Philadelphia, Pennsylvania, USA

SATISH KUMAR, DMD, MDSc, MS
Associate Professor, Periodontics, A.T. Still University, Arizona School of Dentistry and Oral Health, Mesa, Arizona, USA

STEFAN LISTL, DDS, PhD
Professor of Quality and Safety of Oral Health Care, Faculty of Medical Sciences, Radboud University, The Netherlands

PAUL A. MOORE, DMD, PhD, MPH
Professor, Pharmacology and Dental Public Health, University of Pittsburgh School of Dental Medicine, Pittsburgh, Pennsylvania, USA

RICHARD NIEDERMAN, DMD
Professor, Chair, Department of Epidemiology and Health Promotion, New York University College of Dentistry, New York, New York, USA

MARCO A. PERES, BDS, MSc, PhD
Professor of Population Oral Health, Adelaide Dental School, The University of Adelaide, Adelaide, South Australia, Australia

D. BRAD RINDAL, DDS
HealthPartners Institute, Bloomington, Minnesota, USA

JO RYCROFT-MALONE, RN, MSc, PhD
Professor of Health Services Research, Main Arts Building, Bangor University, Bangor, United Kingdom

JOANNA M. SCOTT, PhD
Assistant Professor, Research and Graduate Programs, University of Missouri-Kansas City, School of Dentistry, Kansas City, Missouri, USA

THOMAS P. SOLLECITO, DMD, FDS RCSEd
Professor, Chair of Oral Medicine, University of Pennsylvania School of Dental Medicine, Philadelphia, Pennsylvania, USA

GEORGIOS TSAKOS, BDS, MSc, PhD, FHEA
Reader in Dental Public Health, Department of Epidemiology and Public Health, University College, London, United Kingdom

ROBERT J. WEYANT, MS, DMD, DrPH
Professor and Chair, Department of Dental Public Health, University of Pittsburgh School of Dental Medicine, Pittsburgh, Pennsylvania, USA

Contents

> Constructing an evidence-based dental practice requires leadership, commitment, technology support, and time, as well as skill practice in searching, appraising, and organizing evidence. In mastering the skills of evidence-based dentistry, clinicians can implement high-quality science into practice through a variety of opportunities including the development of clinical care guidelines, procedural technique protocols, and electronic dental record auto-note templates, as well as treatment planning, care prioritization, and case presentation. The benefits of building an evidence-based dental practice are many, including improvements in patient care and satisfaction, increased treatment predictability and confidence in care approaches, as well as potential cost savings.

> Excess added sugars, particularly in the form of sugar-sweetened beverages, is a leading cause of tooth decay in US children. Although added sugar intake is rooted in behavioral and social factors, few evidence-based, theory-driven socio-behavioral strategies are currently available to address added sugar intake. Dental health professionals are in a position to help identify and address problematic sugar-related behaviors in pediatric patients and advocate for broader upstream approaches, including taxes, warning labels, and policy changes, that can help reduce added sugar intake, prevent tooth decay, and improve health outcomes in vulnerable child populations.

> It has been known for centuries that opioids are highly addictive when consumed for prolonged periods of time. Pharmacologic tolerance to the efficacy of opioid analgesic results in a need for increased dosing and drug dependence. One must question the empirical sources of evidence that justified the belief that prescription opioids were safe and effective for treating acute and chronic pain. Progress in developing and applying evidence-based analgesic therapies for acute inflammatory pain is presented.

> This article reviews current evidence on the effectiveness of silver diamine fluoride (SDF) as a caries arresting and preventive agent. It provides

clinical recommendations around SDF's appropriate use as part of a comprehensive caries management program. Systematic reviews confirm that SDF is effective for caries arrest on cavitated lesions in primary teeth and root caries in the elderly. It may also prevent new lesions. Application is easy, noninvasive, affordable, and safe. Although it stains the lesions dark as it arrests them, it provides clinicians with an additional tool for caries management when esthetics are not a primary concern.

This article is an overview to update the practicing general dental practitioner about clinically relevant evidence-based topics published in the recent past in the diagnosis, etiopathogenesis, and management of gingivitis and periodontitis.

Oral medicine is "the discipline of dentistry concerned with the oral health care of medically complex patients, including the diagnosis and primarily nonsurgical treatment and/or management of medically related conditions affecting the oral and maxillofacial region." In each of these areas, evidence-based medicine has shaped theoretic understanding and clinical practice. The available evidence allows for improved patient management. Further evidence, as it becomes available, should be reviewed on a regular basis to guide our clinical practice.

The motivation for teaching evidence-based practice is that, through the use of high-quality clinically relevant evidence, clinicians will make rationale decision that optimally improve patient health outcomes. Achieving that goal requires clinicians who are able to answer patient care–relevant clinical questions efficiently, which means that they must be able rapidly to retrieve, assess, and apply evidence of direct relevance to their patients. Educational programs designed to accomplish this vary in their effectiveness. This article reviews the evidence on educational approaches that may be beneficial when developing educational programs for both dental students and practicing dentists.

The objective of this article was to provide a summary of evidence-based recommendations for the assessment of caries risk and management of dental caries. The goal is to help clinicians manage the caries disease process using personalized interventions supported by the best available evidence, taking into account the clinician's expertise and the patient's needs and preferences, to maintain health and preserve tooth structure.

Significant variation exists in health care practice patterns that creates concerns regarding the quality of care delivered. Clinical practice based on high-quality evidence provides a rationale for clinical decision making. Resources, such as evidence-based guidelines, provide that evidence to clinicians and improve patient outcomes by decreasing unwanted variation in clinical practice. Because knowledge dissemination alone is ineffective to translate scientific evidence into clinical practice, the field of implementation science has emerged to facilitate this translation of research into routine clinical practice. This article provides an introduction to implementation science, and its application in dentistry to promote adoption of evidence-based guidelines.

Generating and implementing evidence-based policy is an important aim for many publicly funded health systems. In dentistry, this is based on the assumption that evidence-based health care increases the efficiency and effectiveness of interventions to improve oral health at a population level. This article argues that a linear logic model that links the generation of research evidence with its use is overly simplistic. It also challenges an uncritical interpretation of the evidence-based paradigm and explores approaches to the evaluation of complex interventions and how they can be embedded into policy and practice to improve oral health at a population level.

DENTAL CLINICS OF NORTH AMERICA

SERIES OF RELATED INTEREST

Atlas of the Oral and Maxillofacial Surgery Clinics
http://www.oralmaxsurgeryatlas.theclinics.com

Oral and Maxillofacial Surgery Clinics
http://www.oralmaxsurgery.theclinics.com

THE CLINICS ARE AVAILABLE ONLINE!
Access your subscription at:
www.theclinics.com

Preface

Evidence-Based Dentistry: The Foundation for Modern Dental Practice

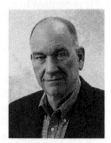

Robert J. Weyant, MS, DMD, DrPH
Editor

Dentistry, as with all branches of medicine, maintains a social contract mandating a professional obligation to adhere to the highest professional standards, ensuring as first principles, that practitioners' decisions and actions are aimed at the well-being and safety of their patients. Meeting this obligation rests in part on ensuring that the decisions about what care is delivered is informed by a thorough understanding of the current best evidence on which approaches to care will provide the best opportunity to realize patient treatment goals.

Unfortunately, it is well documented that there is a substantial gap between what is known about effective health care and what is delivered routinely to patients. The Institute of Medicine characterizes this as the "Know-Do Gap," with the size of that gap reflected in the time lag that occurs between when new evidence on effective treatments becomes available and when that evidence is fully adopted into routine clinical practice.[1]

Unfortunately, this time lag between discovery and adoption of beneficial, evidence-based improvements in patient care often takes years. Why this is so is determined by a complex interaction of factors. These factors include the effectiveness of the dissemination of new evidence, how that evidence is perceived by the dental professional, and the clinical practice environment in which that evidence must be implemented. Evidence dissemination is rapidly improving, as the availability of full text online resources expand. The widespread development of clinical practice guidelines is an important addition to this process and provides an efficient means for translating scientific evidence into clinical practice. The value of clinical guidelines in providing an evidence base for much routine clinical care is emphasized in many of the articles in this issue.

Dent Clin N Am 63 (2019) ix–x
https://doi.org/10.1016/j.cden.2018.09.001
0011-8532/19/© 2018 Published by Elsevier Inc.

Clinical practice can be characterized as uncertain, ambiguous, and constantly changing, consisting of ill-structured problems requiring practical reasoning or professional discretion.[2] However, the best patient outcomes tend to occur when professional discretion is informed by high-quality evidence and not by the dentist's personal preferences, habitual routines, or opinion-driven decisions based on traditional practices.[2] Bringing evidence-based changes into clinical practice is dependent on motivated and well-trained dental professionals who are willing to adopt new approaches to practice and who are operating in an environment that supports (administratively, financially, and technologically) the ability to make those changes. Understanding how to shape the clinical environment to make it receptive to change is the domain of implementation science. The article by Frantsve-Hawley and Rindal provide an overview of the most important issues that must be attended to in this regard. The article by Gillette and Balevi provides details on what is required to construct an evidence-based dental practice. Both articles emphasize the importance of clinical practice guidelines as an efficient means of translating new evidence into routine clinical practice.

At a minimum, effective evidence-based practice (EBP) requires dental professionals to commit to gaining the skills required to find and apply the best available evidence. This requires training in the five-step approach developed by Sackette and Guyette, developed in the 1990s.[3] Their approach is what we now call EBP and is the foundation of the EBP curricula now offered in all health professional schools in the United States. The article by Weyant provides an overview of what is known about effective teaching of EBP and is aimed at guiding EBP trainers in course design as well as dentists who may be selecting an EBP training program.

The overall goal of this issue of the *Dental Clinics of North America* is to provide examples of effective use of evidence and to provide strategies for dentists who wish to increase their use of evidence in routine practice.

Robert J. Weyant, MS, DMD, DrPH
Department of Dental Public Health
University of Pittsburgh School of Dental Medicine
Room 346 Salk Hall
3501 Terrace Street
Pittsburgh, PA 15261, USA

E-mail address:
rjw1@pitt.edu

REFERENCES

1. Institute of Medicine Committee on Quality of Health Care in America. Crossing the quality chasm: a new health system for the 21st century. Washington, DC: National Academy Press; 2001.
2. Algen B. Pedagogical strategies to teach bachelor students evidence-based practice: a systematic review. Nurse Educ Today 2016;36:255–63.
3. Guyatt G, Cairns J, Churchill D, et al, Evidence-Based Medicine Working Group. Evidence-based medicine. A new approach to teaching the practice of medicine. JAMA 1992;268(17):2420–5.

Simple Approaches for Establishing an Evidence-Based Dental Practice

Jane Gillette, DDS, MPH[a],*, Ben Balevi, DDS, MSc[b,c]

KEYWORDS

- Evidence-based practice • Evidence-based dentistry • Clinical care guidelines
- Systematic reviews • Clinical recommendations • Clinical decision making

KEY POINTS

- The benefits of an evidence-based dental practice are improvements in patient care and satisfaction, increased treatment predictability and confidence in care approaches, as well as potential cost savings.
- All dental team members, including nonclinical staff, can play a significant role in establishing an evidence-based dental practice.
- Clinicians can efficiently search and appraise evidence by focusing on evidence-based clinical practice guidelines, Cochrane Reviews, and systematic reviews and primary studies with evidence synopses.
- There are many opportunities for integrating science into practice, including the development of clinical care guidelines, procedural technique protocols, and electronic dental record auto-note templates, as well as treatment planning, care prioritization, and case presentation.

INTRODUCTION

Adopting a commitment to the use of the current best evidence in care delivery is central to ensuring high-quality care and optimal patient outcomes.[1] As with all of medicine, dentistry relies on scientific discovery to advance patient care. In a review of US health care, the Institute of Medicine (IOM) concluded that there were large gaps between the care people *should* receive and the care they *actually* receive.[2] The problem they identified was based on the fact that the translation of new scientific discoveries into routine patient care was a long process fraught with barriers that often lead to

Disclosure Statement: The authors have nothing to disclose.
[a] Sprout Oral Health, PO Box 1028, Bozeman, MT 59771, USA; [b] Private Practice, 805 West Broadway, Suite 306, Vancouver, British Columbia V5Z 1K1, Canada; [c] University of British Columbia, 306-805 West Broadway, Vancouver, British Columbia V5Z 1K1, Canada
* Corresponding author.
E-mail address: drgillette@sproutoralhealth.org

Dent Clin N Am 63 (2019) 1–16
https://doi.org/10.1016/j.cden.2018.08.002
0011-8532/19/© 2018 Elsevier Inc. All rights reserved.

dental.theclinics.com

imperfect application of new knowledge at the point of patient care. The IOM characterized results of this imperfect process in 3 ways. First, they found an overuse of treatments known not to provide patient health benefits. They also found an underuse of treatments known to provide patient health benefits. Finally, they reported routine misuse of treatments such that they failed to deliver their full benefit to patients. They described this problem as the "know-do" gap, meaning that there is frequently a gap between what clinicians know to be best for patients and what care is actually delivered to patients.

Because new knowledge generated from high-quality clinical research often fails to find its way into clinical practice, frontline (dental) health care providers are the focus of much of the efforts of those who create new clinical evidence, as it is frontline providers who ultimately decide whether to adopt and use the science to guide their treatment decisions. The study of the uptake of science into clinical practice is called translational research.

The field of translational research was developed out of the IOM report and similar research documenting the widespread failure across all of health care to consistently apply appropriate new knowledge to improve patient outcomes. The aim of translational research is to address these failures in care delivery by systematically identifying and removing the barriers that prevent new scientific knowledge from being adopted into routine clinical practice. The process of bringing new scientific knowledge to clinical practice is often depicted as a pipeline beginning with basic scientific discoveries and ending with routine patient care, and often referred to as moving knowledge from "bench to bedside" (or in dentistry's case, bench to chairside) (**Fig. 1**).

The focus of this article is the last step in the translational pipeline: the implementation of best available evidence into clinical practice. Specifically, the focus is on the steps needed for a typical dental office to ensure the delivery of optimal oral health care. This process includes the deliberate and systematic selection and application of current best evidence regarding what is known to work and what is known to not work. We call this type of care "best practices." Importantly, the approaches for developing an evidence-based practice, described as follows, empowers the dentists and the office staff to be their own new knowledge producers. This means that the dentist no longer must rely on continuing education courses from "experts" to determine optimal treatment plans. It means that dentists can confidently discuss with patients

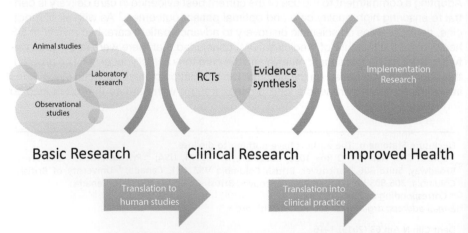

Fig. 1. Translation of research findings from benchtop to chairside. RCTs, randomized controlled trials.

the benefits and harms of any treatment. It also means that a dentist will be confident that they are selected approaches to care that will lead to the best possible outcome for each patient.

APPROACH
Leadership and the Role of the Dental Team

Dentist leaders are uniquely positioned to promote science-based practice through the management of their dental offices and by inspiring and supporting staff in engaging in the evidenced-based dentistry (EBD) process. Organizational mission statements describe to the public the aims and values of a business. One of the largest systemwide impacts can be realized from the development of an organizational mission statement that establishes and defines the practice's commitment to using current best evidence. From the foundation of an organizational commitment to EBD comes a series of systematic strategies and tactics for knitting science into the fabric of a practice. These approaches, which are discussed later, include activities such as the development of Clinical Care Guidelines, treatment planning and prioritization of care, and communicating treatment recommendation to patients. Last, dynamic leadership can motivate and encourage each dental team member to have an active role in cultivating an evidence-based dental practice.[3]

In fact, all members of the dental team, even nonprofessional staff, can be taught a range of skills in EBD. Although advanced training in EBD usually focuses on skill building for dentists and dental hygienists, dental assistants and administrative staff should also have a basic understanding of why evidence-based health care is important, bias and research design, and how to find high-quality and reliable evidence, such as Cochrane Plain Language Summaries. Perfect for dental assistants and administrators, Cochrane US offers a free 6-module online course, *Understanding Evidence-based Healthcare: A Foundation for Action*.[4] Understanding the rationale and framework for science-based care helps promote continuity of messaging to patients throughout the practice, communication of the science-basis for treatment recommendations, and, of course, buy-in related to constructing an EBD practice. This last point is important, as any change in a practice can initially result in more work for staff. Teaching the basics of EBD to support staff helps reinforce the importance of any "extra" work related to the practice change.

Evidence-Based Dentistry Training Resources

At the outset, clinicians may find that they are slower and less accurate in the searching, appraising, summarizing, and organizing of evidence than desired. As with other new skills in dentistry, such as mastering digital impressions, continuing education and repeated practice in EBD skills improves speed and performance. Fortunately, there are many learning opportunities available to practitioners, including in-person courses, online training, journals and books, and study clubs.

Some of the most effective learning happens in educational experiences that include peers, that are in small groups, and in-person. These types of interactions are effective because differing peer perspectives help challenge our own thought processes and beliefs, and peers commonly bring to light questions or topics that may not have been considered otherwise. Specific for dentistry, the American Dental Association (ADA) offers in-person single-day and multiday courses, sometimes in partnership with universities.[5] These courses range from the basic philosophy of EBD, to how to actually conduct systematic reviews (SRs) and meta-analyses. Courses in

EBD also can be found through specialty organizations, such as the American Academy of Pediatric Dentistry, and continuing education programs hosted by national dental organizations and state dental associations.

Looking outside of the profession of dentistry for learning opportunities, such as medicine and nursing, has significant benefits as well. Exposure to other health professions helps broaden and deepen knowledge, not just in terms of evidence-based health care, but working within an interdisciplinary team.[6] For the truly ambitious, 2 universities, McMaster University and Oxford University, offer a range of more intensive options, such as workshops, short courses, and even graduate degrees in evidence-based health care. Basic skill-building workshops, offered at many regional university and public libraries are also useful. Frequently, these classes are no more than an hour long and build practical skills in the use of citation management software, Excel, and literature database searching.

There is a prolific variety of online options available to learners of evidence-based health care (**Box 1**). Online learning, although not interactive, is appealing because of its low cost and convenience. The ADA's Center for Evidence-based Dentistry offers videos and even podcasts specific to dentistry. Another organization, also named the Center for Evidence-based Dentistry but based in the United Kingdom, offers a comprehensive set of resources on question formulation, searching for evidence, and appraising evidence and implementing science into practice. Not specific to dentistry, but science-based practice in general, are numerous online resources, including those from the Center for Evidence-based Medicine (CEBM), Cochrane, and PubMed. The CEBM and Cochrane both have an expansive selection of resources on topics, including interpreting common statics found in SRs, which is usually an area of growth and learning for most clinicians.

For those who prefer the feel of holding a book or a paper, there are many printed materials available, including books, journals, and workbooks (see **Box 1**). A classic book, with detailed, easy-to-understand explanations and examples, is Trisha Greenhalgh's *How to Read a Paper*.[7] This book should be on every EBD learner's list to read. Also, on the must-read-list is the *Journal of the American Dental Association* series on Evidence-based Dentistry.[8] This remarkable series, developed just for the dental profession, is arguably the first EBD learning engagement a clinician should consider. It

---

Box 1
Online and printed evidence-based dentistry learning resources

Online Learning Resources
  The American Dental Association Center for Evidence-based Dentistry (EBD.ADA.org)
  The Centre for Evidence-based Dentistry (cebd.org)
  The Centre for Evidence-based Medicine (cebm.net)
  Cochrane Collaboration (cochrane.org)
  PubMed Tutorials (learn.nlm.nih.gov/documentation/training-packets/T0042010P/)

Printed Learning Resources
  How to Read a Paper[11] (book)
  Critical Thinking: Understanding and Evaluating Dental Research[33] (book)
  Journal of the American Dental Association series on Evidence-based Dentistry (journal manuscripts)
  Evidence-Based Decision Making: a Translational Guide for Dental Professionals[33] (workbook)
  Evidence-Based Dentistry for the Dental Hygienist[33] (workbook)
  Journal of Evidence-based Dental Practice (journal)
  Evidence-based Dentistry (journal)

covers a wide range of topics, including levels of evidence, basic statistics, and appraising and implementing evidence. The strength of this series, besides its comprehensive nature, is that it is written with the dental professional in mind and uses real-world examples and application in dentistry.

Accessing Evidence

Since published scientific evidence is the foundation of EBD, clinicians must have low-cost, easy access to scientific literature. Practitioners usually access low-cost or free health care research in 1 of 2 ways:

1. Through a university medical library (alumni or regional)
2. Through membership in an organization such as the ADA

As a member benefit, the ADA provides free access to a vast number of dental journals, including access to full Cochrane Reviews. Even without either of these 2 options, a significant amount of information is available for free, such as the ADA's EBD Clinical Practice Guidelines and Cochrane Review abstracts, some select full Cochrane Reviews, as well critical summaries of primary and secondary literature such as those developed by the Dental Elf. Regardless of how evidence is accessed (library or organizational membership), most searching is conducted online; consequently, a solid Internet connection and laptop or computer are requirements.

Formulating a Question

The most fundamental step in investigating a clinical topic is formulating a focused clinical question. This is because the question formulated drives the search terms, and insufficient search terms lead to inadequate or misleading search results. A good clinical question typically follows the "PICO" format; that is, your question should define the *Patient/Population, Intervention, Comparison/Control,* and *Intervention.*[9] For example, a sufficient clinical question would be "Do perioperative antibiotics reduce implant failure in adults?" A search strategy that included only the words "dental implants" would result in too many nonrelevant returned results. A search strategy that included the words "amoxicillin prescribed before dental implant placement in the disabled elderly" would be too narrow and not return enough results. Instead, better search terms on this topic would be "antibiotic prophylaxis AND dental implant failure" or "perioperative antibiotics AND dental implants." These 2 approaches would likely capture an adequate number of relevant results.

Finding Evidence

Search approach 1: access evidence-based clinical practice guidelines and systematic reviews with evidence synopses

Because evidence can be stratified according to its level of objectivity and reliability,[10] clinicians should always begin the search process by querying the highest level of evidence. Specifically, this means searching for "secondary" forms of evidence, such as evidence-based clinical practice guidelines (CPGs) and high-quality SRs with evidence synopses (**Table 1**). We strongly advise practitioners attempt this approach first, as this method results in the highest-quality and most meaningful science in the shortest amount of time.

Evidence-based CPGs are care recommendation statements intended to optimize patient health outcomes and include an assessment of both the benefits and harms of the various care options.[11] The process of developing an evidence-based CPG is quite rigorous and costly, often spanning many months to even a year. According to standards for the development of evidence-based CPGs, to be trustworthy, guidelines

Table 1	
EBD resources by evidence type	
Name of Resource	**Type of Evidence**
ADA Center for Evidence-based Dentistry (EBD.ADA.org)	Evidence-based CPG
TRIP Database (tripdatabase.com)	Evidence-based CPG Evidence synopses Systematic reviews Primary studies
PubMed Clinical Queries (ncbi.nlm.nih.gov/pubmed/clinical)	Systematic reviews
Dental Elf (nationalelfservice.net/dentistry/)	Evidence synopses
ADA Library and Archives (ada.org/en/member-center/ada-library)	Full access to Cochrane Reviews and all dental journals, including *Journal of Evidence-based Dental Practice* and *Evidence-based Dentistry* (free to ADA members)
Journal of the American Dental Association: Clinical Scans (jada.ada.org/clinicalscans)	Evidence synopses (free to ADA members)
Journal of Evidence-based Dental Practice	Evidence synopses
Evidence-based Dentistry	Evidence synopses
Cochrane Database of Systematic Reviews (cochranelibrary.com/cochrane-database-of-systematic-reviews/)	Systematic reviews

Abbreviations: ADA, American Dental Association; CPG, clinical practice guideline; EBD, evidence-based dentistry.

should be developed by a multidisciplinary panel of experts and stakeholders, with full disclosure of any potential conflict of interest and transparency of methods and processes used. The guideline must address a clear and specific clinical question, and consider all reasonable options for alternative care. It is essential that the guideline is based on a recent SR to ensure that all evidence regarding risks, harms, benefits, and associated costs are considered. Finally, the guideline must grade the strength of the evidence based on an explicit and standardized approach, such as Grading of Recommendation Assessment Development and Evaluation (GRADE).[12]

An SR is a transparent, structured, and comprehensive process for ensuring that all relevant studies, both published and nonpublished, on a particular clinical question are captured. An SR includes a focused clinical question and a detailed description of how the investigators searched and selected studies for inclusion. If possible, the SR will combine statically the quantitative outcome data from the included individual studies. This process, which is called "meta-analysis," provides readers with a pooled effect estimate of the intervention. SRs, which include meta-analyses based on well-conducted studies, have a low risk of bias and are the best estimate of clinical reality.

Even though evidence-based CPGs and SRs are recognized for their high reliability and comprehensive nature, these forms of science can still differ in quality. Accordingly, a structured, critical evaluation of their quality is important. Evidence synopses are short summary narratives, which include a critical evaluation of the quality of the methods and risk of bias. Most commonly, they are 1 page and authored by an individual with advanced knowledge and expertise in study design and research methods.

The process of evaluating a study's rigor and reliability is called "critical appraisal," and is an essential component of the EBD process. Critical appraisal is a skill that takes knowledge in clinical research methods and basic statistics. Like other skills, it takes time and practice to become proficient. Furthermore, this component of the EBD process takes time to complete. Fortunately, practitioners, even with novice skills in critical appraisal, can both evaluate a study's rigor and applicability of results, and save time in EBD process by focusing on accessing evidence-based CPGs and SRs with evidence synopses (see **Table 1**). Accordingly, focusing on these 2 types of evidence is the strategy for *Search Approach One*. The steps of this approach are depicted in **Fig. 2**.

The 2 best comprehensive resources for finding evidence-based CPGs and SRs with evidence synopses are the Turning Research into Practice "TRIP" Database and the Clinical Queries feature in PubMed. TRIP provides readers with many levels of evidence, including evidence synopses on their topic of interest, whereas the PubMed Clinical Queries feature completes an automatic search that focuses on SRs. Evidence synopses associated with SRs in PubMed are found linked to the bottom of the abstract in the "comment in" section.

Search approach 2: access primary studies with evidence synopses and high-quality systematic reviews

There may be times when neither an evidence-based CPG or an SR with an evidence synopsis exists. In these instances, clinicians should access primary studies with evidence synopses and/or high-quality SRs. As with secondary forms of evidence (CPGs and SRs), primary studies (clinical trials and observational studies) can vary in quality as well. Luckily, many of the evidence synopses resources mentioned previously also include critical summaries for primary literature (**Fig. 3**).

Cochrane Reviews are considered to be the "gold standard" of SRs. As with other SRs, it is possible to find an associated evidence synopsis, which in turn allows the clinician to eliminate the critical appraisal process. However, sometimes there may be a Cochrane Review of interest that does not have an associated synopsis. In this case, a practitioner has 1 of 2 choices. The first option is to skip the critical appraisal process. Due to rigor and precision of Cochrane Reviews, some clinicians elect to omit

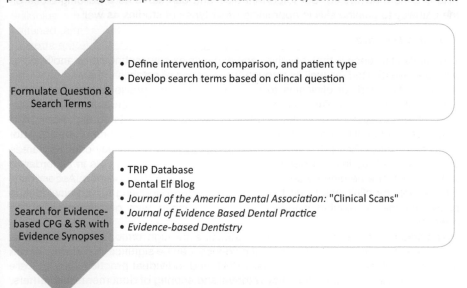

Fig. 2. Search approach 1: access evidence-based CPGs and SRs with evidence synopses.

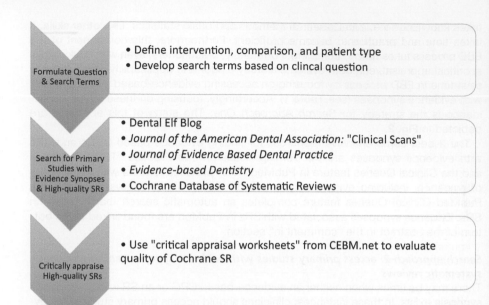

Fig. 3. Search approach 2: access primary studies with evidence synopses and high-quality SRs.

the critical appraisal process when a Cochrane Review is found on their topic of interest.[13] The second option is for clinicians to complete the critical appraisal themselves. Because critical appraisal of scientific studies is a new skill for many, in the beginning it is best to use a structured worksheet designed for this process. The CEBM offers several tools designed for this purpose. Learning to evaluate the quality and bias of SRs is a more advanced, but important skill, and can serve as a building block on the pathway to gaining skill in appraising other types of studies as well.

Managing Evidence

The nature of science is that it evolves and expands as new technologies and hypotheses are investigated, as well as through the retesting of established paradigms. This results in the need for clinicians to monitor and update previously appraised and implemented evidence. There are some topics in dentistry, such as dental sealants, in which the magnitude of effect and the quality of evidence is so significant, that new research is unlikely to change the existing CPGs.[14,15] As such, there may not be as many new SRs on these types of topics. However, in quickly changing areas of science, such as implant dentistry, there is a need to update SRs in accordance with the rate of emerging evidence and the relevance of the question. Accordingly, it is sensible for clinicians to do the same and plan on updating topic knowledge in pace with the developing evidence and/or in concert with germaneness of the question.

The volume of literature that can accumulate through critically appraising evidence, and the regular updating of that evidence, can be significant. Careful citation and document management (ie, SRs, CPGs, and individual practice Clinical Care Guidelines) is important for the easy retrieval and sharing of documents with others, including staff and colleagues. Fortunately, there are many available technologies to assist in managing citations and scientific documents. Citation managers, including

Mendeley, EndNote, and Zotero, are all popular options. Zotero and Mendeley are open-source, free options. Zotero additionally has an import plug-in that downloads and saves source items, including PDFs, of manuscripts, videos, and Web sites, as well as a convenient tagging feature that allows for quick identification of related articles. All 3 citation managers allow some form of sharing of citations with others.

Cloud-based technology is another mechanism for managing and retrieving evidence. It has the added benefit of low-cost file-sharing with staff and peers. In cloud-based evidence management, separate topic folders and subfolders are created. For instance, a main folder might be created named "Oral and Maxillofacial Surgery," and then separate subfolders created under the main folder named "Implantology," "Third-Molar Removal," "Osteonecrosis," and so on. Individual articles are then saved in each subfolder along with any corresponding practice-specific Clinical Care Guidelines. With respect to file naming, the use of a concise description, plus publication date, will assist with quick file identification and retrieval. For example, a summarizing filename for *A practical approach to evidence-based dentistry: X How to avoid being misled by clinical studies' results in dentistry*, might be "Series on EBD10_JADA_avoid being misled_2015."[16]

Implement Evidence into Clinical Practice

EBD can be integrated easily into clinical care with a small amount of thoughtful planning. Similar to learning and introducing a new surgical procedure into your practice, it takes time to become proficient at EBD, as well as to establish staff buy-in. Setting aside small amounts of quiet, uninterrupted time will help with learning the skills of searching and appraising evidence. As any clinician knows, office changes are dramatically smoother when support staff are invested in the change. Creating staff buy-in will likely require explanatory conversations as to why the changes are necessary, as well as an understanding of the benefits to be gained by both patients and the practice. In the following sections, we discuss various opportunities to incorporate EBD in practice. Some of these techniques involve staff work. Accordingly, it is quite important for the staff to be motivated to engage in that work.

Occasionally, providers will be faced with high-quality evidence that is either contrary to how they or their peers practice or that could lead to decreased revenue to the practice if implemented. The emotional tension that results from holding this conflicting knowledge is called cognitive dissonance.[17] A common reaction to these conflicting thoughts and feelings is to (1) dismiss the new-found science either by minimizing or distorting its significance, (2) find reasons to conclude the study results are false or not applicable, or (3) cherry-pick low-level evidence or use anecdotal evidence to support the current practice. This reaction is understandable. Change is difficult, even without conflicting thoughts and ideas; however, there are a few methods for addressing these conflicting feelings. First, based on the quality of the evidence and typical patient values, write a pro and con list of the current practice and the newly investigated care approach. Evaluate and compare these pros and cons. Second, build professional relationships with other clinicians who have already embraced the new evidence-based approach. They can likely provide advice on how and why they made the transition. Third, learn more about the scientific basis for the care approach. In the end, implementing evidence-based approaches increases treatment predictability (ie, reduces treatment failures) and diminishes the use of ineffective care, which in return can result in significant cost savings and improved patient satisfaction.

There are many opportunities for integrating EBD into clinical care. As with any practice change, such as adding a new dental material, it is best to start small. Our recommendation is to begin with assessing areas of care within the practice that are (1) supported by high-quality evidence and/or (2) common procedures in the practice, such as routine dental prophylaxis, periodic dental examinations, and periodic dental radiographs. With respect to selecting a treatment approach of interest, a clinician, at the end of an evidence search and appraisal process, should be able to confidently answer, to some extent, the following questions:

- What clinical condition does this service treat or prevent?
- What type of patient should receive this service?
- What health benefit does a patient receive from this service and what is the magnitude of that benefit?
- Are there any risks associated with the treatment?
- How often should a patient receive this service and does the interval vary according to disease risk status?

Treatment planning, including prioritization of care, and case presentation present additional opportunities for incorporating EBD into practice. Scientific findings can be used to make clinical decisions, such as the appropriate restorative material to use (ie, amalgam vs composite),[18] whether to use adjunct interventions with nonsurgical periodontal therapy (ie, subantimicrobial dose doxycycline),[19] or whether to complete a root canal treatment in 1 or 2 visits.[20] Magnitude of effect can be used to prioritize care. For example, due to the magnitude of the effectiveness of dental sealants,[21] a pediatric dental office might consider scheduling children for a dental examination and dental sealants, instead of a dental examination and routine dental prophylaxis. Finally, distilling the evidence that supports a dental treatment into plain language can help communicate to patients why a particular procedure is important and needed. A patient may be hesitant to accept a certain care recommendation, for example, bone grafting after an extraction to preserve alveolar ridge height,[22] but sharing the science basis for this approach can help a patient feel more confident with the recommendation.

Some practices integrate high-quality science into Clinical Care Guidelines and electronic dental record chart auto-note templates. Clinical Care Guidelines are formal written documents that summarize the evidence and resulting treatment approach for the particular topic of interest. These written documents are shared with the entire dental team and used to guide care throughout the office. This not only promotes the efficient continuity of care, but also helps reduce errors that could result in harm to the patient (**Box 2**). Once Clinical Care Guidelines are established for the practice, they can be incorporated into electronic dental record chart auto-note templates. For example, a practice may develop a Clinical Care Guideline on Peri-Procedural Management of Patients on Anticoagulant Therapy[23] and then embed a quick reference to the guideline in the chart auto-note template which reads "Evidence does not support modification of anticoagulant therapy before dental extraction (Nishimura, 2014)." This approach has 3 distinct benefits. First, auto-embedding reference to the guideline saves time over hand-typing and entry. Second, referencing the high-level evidence helps reduce legal risk exposure in the event of an adverse event. Finally, citing the scientific rationale for care can provide protection in the event of an insurance or Medicaid audit.

Being surgeons, most dentists will of course be interested in surgical procedural techniques. There are many technical questions that are of interest to dentists, such as "What is the most accurate and predictable technique for picking the shade of

---

Box 2
Practice guideline hometown dental clinic: management of patients with prosthetic joints undergoing dental procedures

Background: There are over 1 million joint replacements completed annually in the US.[24] Historically, antibiotics have been prescribed before dental procedures for patients with prosthetic joints with the intent of avoiding prosthetic joint infection (PJI). However, synthesized high-quality evidence does not support this practice. A recent clinical guideline developed by the America Dental Association based on systematic review[25] notes:

- There is evidence that dental procedures are not associated with prosthetic joint implant infections.

- There is evidence that antibiotics provided before oral care do not prevent prosthetic joint implant infections.

- There are potential harms of antibiotics including risk for anaphylaxis, antibiotic resistance, and opportunistic infections like *Clostridium difficile.*

- The benefits of antibiotic prophylaxis may not exceed the harms for most patients.

- The individual patient's circumstances and preferences should be considered when deciding whether to prescribe prophylactic antibiotics prior to dental procedures.

Therefore, it is the clinical practice of Hometown Dental Clinic to not routinely prescribe antibiotics prior to dental procedures for patients with prosthetic joint implants for the prevention of PJI. Though routine prescribing of antibiotics before undergoing dental procedures with gingival manipulation or mucosal incision is not advised, some limited populations may benefit from antibiotic prophylaxis including those with a history of drainage or infection after undergoing arthroplasty. As always, providers should acquire a complete health history and review a patient's medical status thoroughly when making final decisions regarding the need for antibiotic prophylaxis.

---

an anterior porcelain crown?" or "Do I always need to cut my preparation with water or are there times when I can cut the preparation dry?" Many of these topics have a paucity of high-quality studies to support them. In fact, the *Journal of the American Dental Association* routinely publishes case presentations of treatment and surgical techniques for this very reason. Nevertheless, there are some instances in which techniques are highlighted by noteworthy science. For example, a 2014 Cochrane Systematic Review considered, among other treatment approaches, the best flap design to reduce dry socket.[26] A 2016 systematic review published in the *Journal of Prosthodontics* considered different approaches for gingival retraction that minimize adverse effects to gum health, a topic that is very important when considering anterior esthetics.[27]

Finally, comparing the evidence for effectiveness and magnitude of effectiveness between 2 treatments in relation to the cost of the 2 treatments can result in cost savings to both the practice and the patient as well. New dental technologies and therapies emerge as quickly as the cost of those technologies rise. Accordingly, it becomes vitally important to critically consider each new technology purchase for the practice. Sometimes a new technology is significantly better than the old technology; sometimes it is not. SRs that include clinical trials that compare the "gold standard" technology to new technologies can be helpful in assisting dental practitioners to determine whether the new approach is worth the investment. For example, a 2017 *Evidence-based Clinical Practice Guideline for the Evaluation of Potentially Malignant Disorders in the Oral Cavity* concluded that autofluorescence technology of innocuous lesions is not advised due the very high false-positive rate and the availability of more predicable screening tools.[28] Considering the evidence of effectiveness and the cost of that technology ($4000), compared with effective traditional oral cancer manual/visual screening, autofluorescence technology may not be worth the practice investment.

SUMMARY

The process of setting up and engaging fully in an evidence-based dental practice takes leadership, commitment, preparation, and time. The section "Putting It All Together—A Case Study: The Prevention of Dry Socket" demonstrates this process, and how a clinician can efficiently search, and implement into care, the high-quality science contained within SRs and summarized and appraised with evidence synopses. For the patient, and the clinician, there are many benefits, including improvements in patient care and satisfaction, increased treatment predictability and confidence in care approaches, as well as potential cost savings. In the end, the skills, training, and resources needed to routinely engage in evidence-based care are minimal compared with the improvements in quality of care that patients receive, and deserve.

Putting it all together—a case study: the prevention of dry socket

Dr Johnston, the dental director of a multidentist community health center (CHC) dental clinic, was having lunch with his colleague, when his friend announced she had begun using chlorhexidine gluconate 0.12% (CHX) for intrasocket irrigation to prevent dry socket (alveolar osteitis). The next day at work, Dr Johnston began to think about this approach and wondered if the technique might be a care approach his clinic should implement. With use of reports from the clinic's electronic dental record, Dr Johnston was able to determine that on average 50 middle-aged adults had 1 or more third molars extracted each month. Due to the clinic's use of dental diagnostic codes, he was able to assess that most third-molar extractions were due to periodontal disease, caries, pulpal pathology, and/or nonrestorability, and that approximately 14% of patients receiving third-molar extraction required postoperative follow-up care.

Before reviewing the evidence, Dr Johnston formulated his search terms and a set of questions to answer, including the following:

- In an adult population, are there local interventions (such as intrasocket irrigation with CHX) that prevent dry socket?
- Search terms: alveolar osteitis AND chlorhexidine
- What is the magnitude of these effects?
- What is the level of confidence in the science?
- What is the cost of the intervention to the CHC?
- Are there any harms?
- Should the CHC implement the practice in the form of a clinic-wide Clinical Care Guideline?

Searching

Dr Johnston searched the TRIP database, but did not find any evidence-based CPGs. He then searched the Clinical Queries section of PubMed and found 2 SRs, which also had critical summaries associated with them. He found a 2012 Cochrane SR[29] with a critical summary published in *Evidence-based Dentistry*[30] and a 2017 SR[31] with a critical summary published in the *Journal of the American Dental Association* (JADA).[32] He saved these 4 citations to a PubMed "clipboard" (**Figs. 4** and **5**).

Because Dr Johnston was a member of the ADA, he logged into his ADA account and accessed the ADA Library and Archives. There he downloaded the full 2012 Cochrane SR and the critical summary of the SR published in *Evidence-based Dentistry.* He additionally downloaded the 2017 SR published in the *Journal of Oral and Maxillofacial Surgery.* Accessing JADA directly through his online ADA membership account, Dr Johnston downloaded the critical summary of the 2017 SR.

Saving and Organizing

Within Zotero, Dr Johnston created a subcollection (folder) named "Dry Socket Prevention" in his major collection (folder) named "Oral Surgery." As he accessed the 4 citations in PubMed, he auto-uploaded the citation information into Zotero using the program's import feature. He added the downloaded articles as files to the Zotero citations. In this process, Zotero automatically created tags for each article.

Appraising and Summarizing the Evidence

Assessing the quality of the SRs and the summarizing the evidence was actually fairly easy for Dr Johnston, because each SR had its own critical summary. What Dr Johnston found was that both SRs used recognized review methods and were of high quality. Encouragingly, each review reported similar findings, that CHX, either as a pre and post rinse or as a gel placed in the socket after surgery, reduced the occurrence of dry socket. There were no trials included in either of the reviews that evaluated the effectiveness of intrasocket irrigation. The CHX rinse was already stocked in his clinic and the CHX gel was not available for him to purchase, so he decided to focus on literature describing CHX rinsing.

If a high prevalence of dry socket (30%) was assumed, both studies reported that a clinician would need to treat 8 patients with a CHX rinse (before and after surgery) to prevent 1 case of dry socket. The Cochrane SR further clarified that if a more modest prevalence of dry socket was assumed (5%) that 47 patients would need to receive CHX to prevent 1 case of dry socket.

Risk of Harm and Cost

With respect to adverse reactions, the studies reported staining and altered taste as the most common risks. Dr Johnston also searched the US Food and Drug Administration (FDA) Web site, where he found an FDA drug warning for CHX that reported rare but serious life-threatening allergies to CHX.[33]

He then logged into his dental supply vendor Web site and found the cost for one 16-oz bottle of CHX to be approximately $13.00. Patients before and after rinsing with CHX would use approximately 1 oz total (0.5 oz before surgery and 0.5 oz after surgery). Accordingly, 1 bottle could be used to treat 16 patients or approximately $0.80 per patient.

Implementation

The background section of the Cochrane SR noted that dry sockets are most common in the fourth decade of life and can be associated with infection around the tooth to be extracted, inadequate oral hygiene, poor postsurgical care, and smoking. Between these reported risk factors, which matched his clinic population, and the internal clinic data, which reported approximately 14% of patients required a postoperative follow-up, Dr Johnston concluded that the prevalence of dry socket at his clinic was likely approximately 20%. Based on the number needed to treat data reported in the SRs, he predicted that clinicians would need to treat approximately 12 patients with CHX to prevent 1 case of dry socket. Dr Johnston believed this to be clinically significant.

Accordingly, Dr Johnston developed a Clinical Care Guideline on the Prevention of Dry Socket. At the bottom of the Clinical Care Guideline Document he notated that the guideline should be updated in 3 years. During a whole-staff monthly meeting, Dr Johnston presented the science, the supporting technique, and new Clinical Care Guideline to be implemented across the clinic. He instructed the staff to use the ICD-10 diagnosis code M27.3 (alveolitis of jaws) for any postoperative appointments in which a patient was treated for dry socket, as this would allow for more precise monitoring of dry socket rates in the clinic. To address the rare but potentially serious harm of CHX allergy, he made sure that all staff were adequately trained to identify the signs and symptoms of an anaphylactic allergy and be prepared to respond quickly to this type of medical emergency.

Over the next year, Dr Johnston monitored the rate of postoperative returns due to dry socket with use of the new diagnostic code. He found that in fact the rate of postoperative returns for dry socket dropped from 14% to 8% (7 per month to 4 per month). The extra 3 appointments saved per month were used to care for other clinic patients with treatment needs. The revenue from these 3 additional patient care visits more than covered the cost of implementing the new CHX rinsing protocol.

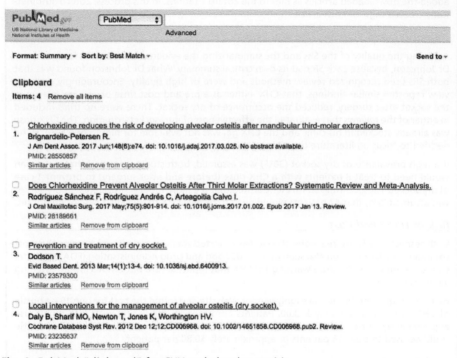

Fig. 4. PubMed "clipboard" for CHX and alveolar osteitis.

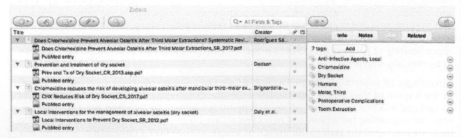

Fig. 5. Zotero management of citations and science documents. *Courtesy of* Roy Rosenzweig Center for History and New Media, Fairfax, VA.

REFERENCES

1. Niederman R, Richards D, Brands W. The changing standard of care. J Am Dent Assoc 2012;143(5):434–7.
2. Corrigan, Janet M. Crossing the quality chasm: a new health system for the 21st century. Washington, DC: National Academy Press; 2009.
3. Frideres T, Gillette J. Evidence-based dentistry professional development and training for the dental office team. J Evid Based Dent Pract 2009;9(3):129–34.
4. Cochrane United States. Understanding evidence-based healthcare: a foundation for action | Cochrane United States. Available at: http://us.cochrane.org/understanding-evidence-based-healthcare-foundation-action. Accessed July 5, 2018.
5. Educational Courses. American Dental Association. Available at: EBD.ADA.org; https://ebd.ada.org/en/education/courses. Accessed July 1, 2018.
6. Weintraub J. What should oral health professionals know in 2040: executive summary. J Dent Educ 2017;81(08):1024–32.
7. Greenhalgh T. How to read a paper: the basics of evidence-based medicine. Chichester (England): John Wiley & Sons; 2014.
8. Brignardello-Petersen R, Carrasco-Labra A, Glick M, et al. A practical approach to evidence-based dentistry. J Am Dent Assoc 2014;145(11):1105–7.
9. Brignardello-Petersen R, Carrasco-Labra A, Booth HA, et al. A practical approach to evidence-based dentistry. J Am Dent Assoc 2014;145(12):1262–7.
10. Levels of Evidence. Oxford Center for Evidence-based Medicine. Available at: www.cebm.net/2009/06/oxford-centre-evidence-based-medicine-levels-evidence-march-2009/. Accessed July 1, 2018.
11. Graham R. Clinical practice guidelines we can trust. Washington, DC: National Academies Press; 2011.
12. Atkins D, Best D, Briss PA, et al. Grading quality of evidence and strength of recommendations. BMJ 2004;328(7454):1490.
13. Useem J, Brennan A, Lavalley M, et al. Systematic differences between Cochrane and non-Cochrane meta-analyses on the same topic: a matched pair analysis. PLoS One 2015;10(12):e0144980.
14. Takwoingi Y, Hopewell S, Tovey D, et al. A multicomponent decision tool for prioritising the updating of systematic reviews. BMJ 2013;347:f7191.
15. When and how to update systematic reviews: consensus and checklist. BMJ 2016;354:i4853.
16. Carrasco-Labra A, Brignardello-Petersen R, Azarpazhooh A, et al. A practical approach to evidence-based dentistry: X. J Am Dent Assoc 2015;146(12):919–24.
17. Tavris C, Aronson E. Mistakes were made (but not by me): why we justify foolish beliefs, bad decisions and hurtful acts. London: Pinter & Martin; 2016.
18. Afrashtehfar KI, Emami E, Ahmadi M, et al. Failure rate of single-unit restorations on posterior vital teeth: a systematic review. J Prosthet Dent 2017;117(3):345–53.e8.
19. Smiley CJ, Tracy SL, Abt E, et al. Evidence-based clinical practice guideline on the nonsurgical treatment of chronic periodontitis by means of scaling and root planing with or without adjuncts. J Am Dent Assoc 2015;146(7):525–35.
20. Manfredi M, Figini L, Gagliani M, et al. Single versus multiple visits for endodontic treatment of permanent teeth. Cochrane Database Syst Rev 2016;(12):CD005296.

21. Wright JT, Crall JJ, Fontana M, et al. Evidence-based clinical practice guideline for the use of pit-and-fissure sealants: a report of the American Dental Association and the American Academy of Pediatric Dentistry. J Am Dent Assoc 2016; 147(8):672–82.e12.
22. Avila-Ortiz G, Elangovan S, Kramer K, et al. Effect of alveolar ridge preservation after tooth extraction. J Dent Res 2014;93(10):950–8.
23. Nishimura RA, Otto CM, Bonow RO, et al. 2017 AHA/ACC focused update of the 2014 AHA/ACC guideline for the management of patients with valvular heart disease: a report of the American College of Cardiology/American Heart Association Task Force on clinical practice guidelines. Circulation 2017;135(25):e1159–95.
24. Hospital Utilization (in non-Federal short-stay hospitals). Centers for Disease Control and Prevention. Available at: https://cdc.gov/nchs/fastats/inpatient-surgery.htm. Published June 2, 2009. Accessed September 16, 2018.
25. Sollecito TP, Abt E, Lockhart PB, et al. The use of prophylactic antibiotics prior to dental procedures in patients with prosthetic joints. The Journal of the American Dental Association 2015;146(1).
26. Coulthard P, Bailey E, Esposito M, et al. Surgical techniques for the removal of mandibular wisdom teeth. Cochrane Database Syst Rev 2014;(7):CD004345.
27. Tabassum S, Adnan S, Khan FR. Gingival retraction methods: a systematic review. J Prosthodont 2016;26(8):637–43.
28. Lingen MW, Abt E, Agrawal N, et al. Evidence-based clinical practice guideline for the evaluation of potentially malignant disorders in the oral cavity: a report of the American Dental Association. J Am Dent Assoc 2017;148(10):712–27.e10.
29. Daly B, Sharif MO, Newton T, et al. Local interventions for the management of alveolar osteitis (dry socket). Cochrane Database Syst Rev 2012;(12):CD006968.
30. Dodson T. Prevention and treatment of dry socket. Evid Based Dent 2013;14(1): 13–4.
31. Sánchez FR, Andrés CR, Calvo IA. Does chlorhexidine prevent alveolar osteitis after third molar extractions? Systematic review and meta-analysis. J Oral Maxillofac Surg 2017;75(5):901–14.
32. Brignardello-Petersen R. Chlorhexidine reduces the risk of developing alveolar osteitis after mandibular third-molar extractions. J Am Dent Assoc 2017;148(6): e74.
33. FDA Drug Safety Communication: FDA warns about rare but serious allergic reactions with the skin antiseptic chlorhexidine gluconate. Available at: fda.gov; https://www.fda.gov/Drugs/DrugSafety/ucm530975.htm. Accessed July 1, 2018.

Added Sugar and Dental Caries in Children
A Scientific Update and Future Steps

Donald L. Chi, DDS, PhD[a],*, JoAnna M. Scott, PhD[b]

KEYWORDS

- Added sugars • Sugar-sweetened beverages • Dental caries • Children
- Pediatric dentistry • Evidence-based dentistry • Behavioral determinants of health
- Social determinants of health

KEY POINTS

- Added sugar intake is strongly associated with tooth decay in US children.
- Sugar-sweetened beverages are the main source of added sugars. Health education is necessary but insufficient in improving beverage behaviors.
- Social factors like socioeconomic disadvantage, household habits, and availability through local stores influence added sugar intake.
- Socio-behavioral interventions are relatively uncommon but are a promising approach in reducing added sugar intake and preventing tooth decay in children.
- Upstream approaches like sugar-sweetened beverage bans in schools, warning labels, and taxes can further reduce excess added sugar intake.

INTRODUCTION

Dental caries is the most common disease globally and among US children.[1,2] The causal relationship between fermentable carbohydrates and caries was first documented in the scientific literature in the 1950s. The Vipeholm study underscored the importance of both frequency of sugar intake and the consistency of sugar consumed.[3–6] Until this landmark set of publications, there was no scientific consensus on the link between sugar and caries.[4] It is now widely accepted that

Disclosure Statement: The study was funded by U.S. National Institute of Dental and Craniofacial Research (NIDCR), R56DE025813 and the William T. Grant Foundation Scholars Program.
[a] Department of Oral Health Sciences, University of Washington, School of Dentistry, Box 357475, B509 Health Sciences Building, Seattle, WA 98195-7475, USA; [b] Research and Graduate Programs, University of Missouri Kansas City, School of Dentistry, 650 E. 25th Street, Kansas City, MO 64108, USA
* Corresponding author.
E-mail address: dchi@uw.edu

Dent Clin N Am 63 (2019) 17–33
https://doi.org/10.1016/j.cden.2018.08.003
dental.theclinics.com

excess intake of added sugars, defined as sugars found in foods other than grains, vegetables, whole fruit, and milk, leads to dental caries and other systemic health problems, including obesity, diabetes, and cardiovascular diseases.[7–10]

Despite decades of research on sugar as one of the main causes of dental caries, there are currently few evidence-based clinical strategies known to reduce excess added sugar intake in children.[11] The goal of this article is to present national data on the relationship between added sugar and dental caries in US children; identify the sociodemographic, behavioral, and social determinants of added sugar intake in children; review evidence-based strategies that reduce added sugar intake; provide clinicians with chairside strategies to address excess added sugar intake in patients; and outline unresolved challenges, opportunities, and next steps. The intent of this review is to advance the field through promotion of high-quality, evidence-based strategies and policies that address added sugar intake in children, which in turn are expected to prevent oral and systemic diseases, reduce health inequalities, improve quality of life, and address other consequences related to excess added sugar intake.

Added Sugar and Dental Caries

Based on data from the 2011 to 2012 US National Health and Nutrition Examination Survey (NHANES), there is a positive and statistically significant relationship between added sugar intake (grams per day) and dental caries (defined as the number of decayed, missing, or filled primary and permanent tooth surfaces as a proportion of the total number of tooth surfaces in the mouth) for children aged 18 years and younger (**Fig. 1**). Although these data are cross-sectional and do not account for longitudinal or accumulated sugar intake, the noted relationship is consistent with the sugar-mediated pathobiology of dental caries.[12]

Sociodemographic Determinants

There are 4 sociodemographic determinants relevant in added sugar intake.[13] The first is age. Based on 2011 to 2012 NHANES data for US children aged 18 years and

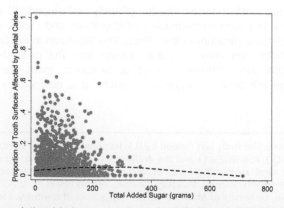

Fig. 1. Plot of mean daily added sugar intake and tooth decay for US children aged 18 years and younger (N = 3441). Plot not adjusted for potential outliers. (*Data from* National Center for Health Statistics. 2011–2012 U.S. National Health and Nutrition Examination Survey (NHANES) data for participants ages 18 years and younger with added sugar and caries data. Available at: https://wwwn.cdc.gov/nchs/nhanes/ContinuousNhanes/Default.aspx?BeginYear=2011. Accessed June 1, 2018.)

younger with complete data on added sugar intake and dental caries (N = 3441), added sugar intake increases with age (**Fig. 2**). Added sugar intake ranged from 3.5 g per day for children younger than 1 year to 102.1 g per day for children aged 18 years. Added sugar intake is significantly lower for children younger than 6 years than for children aged 6 to 18 years. These data are consistent with findings from other studies examining age-based trends in added sugar intake.[14]

The second sociodemographic determinant is race and ethnicity. Added sugar intake was highest for non-Hispanic white children aged 18 years and younger (80.3 g) compared with nonwhite children (*P*<.05 for all comparisons) based on 2011 to 2012 NHANES data (**Fig. 3**). Added sugar intake for non-Hispanic black, Hispanic, other/multiple race, and Asian children was 72.2, 65.4, 57.4, 51.1 g per day, respectively. Consistent with these data are findings from a study comparing added sugar intake for black and Hispanic children enrolled in the Special Supplemental Nutrition Program for Women, Infants, and Children (WIC) in Chicago.[15] Calories from added sugar intake were significantly higher for black children than for Hispanic children (*P*<.01). A study focusing on American Indian preschoolers found that mean added sugar intake for children aged 2 to 3 years and children 4 to 5 years was 54.8 and 59.1 g, respectively.[16] Added sugar intake was measured using 24-hour recalls. Using NHANES data as a historical comparison group, added sugar intake was 17.5% greater for American Indians than intake for white children aged 2 to 3 years but 13.3% lower for American Indians compared with white children aged 4 to 5 years. Another study of Alaska Native children aged 6 to 17 years reported a mean daily added sugar intake of 193 g per day.[17] Added sugar was measured using a hair biomarker validated against 24-hour recalls. Added sugar intake for Alaska Native children was double the mean added sugar intake for white children aged 6 to 17 years in NHANES.

The third sociodemographic factor is income. The relationship between income and added sugar intake is curvilinear, increasing from the lowest-income households to

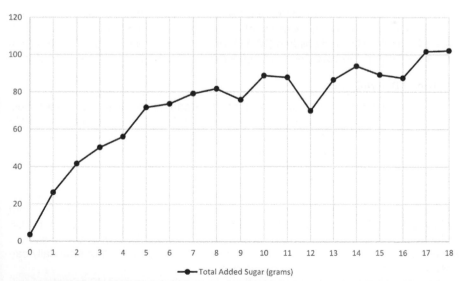

Fig. 2. Mean daily added sugar intake by age group for US children aged 18 years and younger (N = 3441). (*Data from* National Center for Health Statistics. 2011–2012 U.S. National Health and Nutrition Examination Survey (NHANES) data for participants ages 18 years and younger with added sugar and caries data. Available at: https://wwwn.cdc.gov/nchs/nhanes/ContinuousNhanes/Default.aspx?BeginYear=2011. Accessed June 1, 2018.)

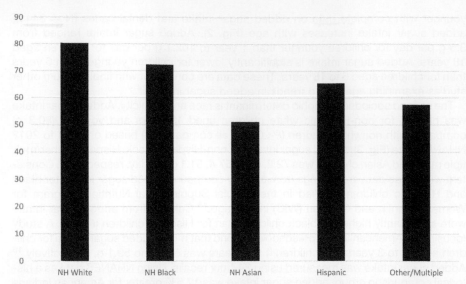

Fig. 3. Mean daily added sugar intake (grams) by race and ethnicity for US children aged 18 years and younger (N = 3441). NH, non-Hispanic. (*Data from* National Center for Health Statistics. 2011–2012 U.S. National Health and Nutrition Examination Survey (NHANES) data for participants ages 18 years and younger with added sugar and caries data. Available at: https://wwwn.cdc.gov/nchs/nhanes/ContinuousNhanes/Default.aspx?BeginYear=2011. Accessed June 1, 2018.)

category 3, then decreasing among children from the highest-income households (**Fig. 4**). Only the difference between categories 1 and 3 was statistically significant (*P* = .01).

The fourth sociodemographic factor is health insurance status, a proxy for income. Added sugar intake was highest for children without health insurance (78.9 g/d), lowest for publicly insured children (70.9 g), and intermediate for children with private insurance (74.3 g). However, none of these differences were statistically significant.

Behavioral Determinants

The behavioral determinants of added sugar intake can be classified into 3 categories. The first is added sugar source. Four waves of NHANES data indicated that for US children aged 6 to 11 years and aged 12 to 19 years, carbonated beverages, energy drinks, and sports drinks were the main source of added sugars (13% and 27%, respectively), followed by grain-based desserts (8.7% and 7.2%), fruit drinks (9.6% and 8.1%), ready-to-eat cereals (5.8% and 4.8%), and candies (5.7% and 5.4%).[18] In another study based on 2009 to 2012 NHANES data, sugar-sweetened beverages (defined as carbonated beverages, fruit drinks, sport and energy drinks, but not including 100% fruit juices) were the most common source of added sugars for US children aged 2 to 18 years.[19] Two-thirds of children aged 2 to 18 years consumed at least one sugar-sweetened beverage serving per day, and 7.3% of total daily calories were from sugar-sweetened beverages.[20]

The second is parent beliefs and practices. In an online survey of US parents of children aged 2 to 17 years (N = 982), parent beliefs that sugary fruit drinks are healthy were significantly associated with the purchases of sugary fruit drinks.[21] Another study of parents of children aged 8 to 14 years in Australia (N = 1302) examined parent attitudes about soft drinks.[22] More specifically, attitudes that soft drinks were enjoyable,

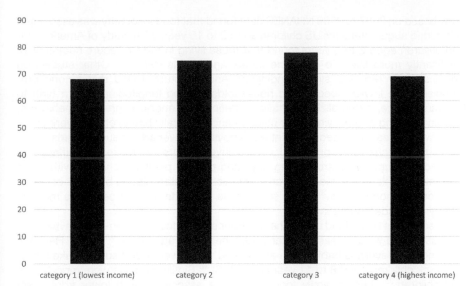

Fig. 4. Mean daily added sugar intake by income category for US children aged 18 years and younger (N = 3441). Income categories calculated as poverty to household income ratio. (*Data from* National Center for Health Statistics. 2011–2012 U.S. National Health and Nutrition Examination Survey (NHANES) data for participants ages 18 years and younger with added sugar and caries data. Available at: https://wwwn.cdc.gov/nchs/nhanes/ContinuousNhanes/Default.aspx?BeginYear=2011. Accessed June 1, 2018.)

tasty, convenient, and a good value were associated with increased intake. Similarly, a qualitative study of Hispanic parents of preschool-aged children (N = 19) reported convenience, cost, and taste as factors related to parents providing children with sugar-sweetened beverages.[23]

The third is child demand and related factors. Parent intake of sugar-sweetened beverages is strongly associated with child intake.[24] Another study found a significant association between child and parent sugar-sweetened beverage intake in African American children aged 3 to 13 years.[25] The previously cited study from Australia found that the frequency of soft drink intake was associated with an increased demand from children for soft drinks they had seen advertised on television.[22] A review of studies on the psychosocial determinants of eating behaviors in children and adolescents identified norms, liking, and preferences as being positively associated with sugar-sweetened beverage intake.[26] Another study of US adolescents aged 12 to 18 years (N = 102) found that adolescents' subjective norms, defined as the extent to which people important to the adolescent want the adolescent to consume less sugary drinks, were associated with intention to limit sugary drinks.[27] A longitudinal observational study of Dutch adolescents aged 12 to 13 years (N = 348) found that high perceived behavioral control was associated with decreased sugar-sweetened beverage intake over a 4-month period in the absence of an intervention.[28] Offering sugary snacks to children aged 5 to 10 years during after-school programs increased intake.[29] Prospectively restricting sweets among Dutch children aged 5 to 7 years led to a desire for sweets that remained high.[30]

Social Determinants

The social determinants of added sugar intake can be classified into 4 categories. The first is socioeconomic disadvantage, for which there are several proxy variables. A study based on 2007 to 2009 NHANES data found that food insecurity was associated with added sugar intake for US children aged 2 to 15 years.[31] A study of American Indian children aged 2 to 5 years found that those living in food-insecure homes were significantly more likely to consume sodas and sports drinks.[32] Other studies on food insecurity reported similar findings.[33] Another study found that among preschoolers from low-socioeconomic households studied longitudinally from birth to 14 years of age, externalizing behaviors (defined as angry, aggressive behaviors, including fighting and bullying other children and physically hitting others) were associated with increased added sugar intake in boys but lower added sugar in girls.[34] Hypothesized mechanisms proposed by the investigators for these sex differences included low impulse control among boys and parents pacifying children with foods differentially. This age is the time frame at which girls start dieting because of media influences on body image.[35] It is also possible that externalizing behaviors mediate poverty and added-sugar intake.[36]

The second is household dietary habits. Four studies found that in-home availability was associated with increased sugar-sweetened beverage intake.[23,25,28,37] Healthier snacking and beverage habits were associated with lower added sugar intake for urban black children aged 8 to 11 years (N = 126).[38] Similar findings were reported for rural children.[39] Stricter family food rules were associated with lower adolescent sugar-sweetened beverage intake.[28]

The third is location of the added sugar source. A 2014 study compared places where children aged 2 to 18 years obtained added sugars using 2009 to 2010 US NHANES data.[40] Stores were the most common source of sugar-sweetened beverages, compared with schools and fast food restaurants. Another study found that introducing a full-scale supermarket in a former food desert reduced added sugar intake.[41] Corner stores were a common source of sugary beverages for children.[42]

The fourth is peer influence. A study from the United States found that adolescent sugar-sweetened beverage intake was significantly associated with peer intake.[43] A prospective study of 141 Dutch children (mean age: 7.7 ±1.3 years) found that a peer modeling intervention involving photos, video clips, and interactive activities instructing children not to follow other peers' food intake behaviors significantly reduced candy intake.[44]

Evidence-Based Strategies

There are several evidence-based strategies that reduce added sugar intake. A 2015 systematic review concluded that interventions involving physical access to sugary beverage alternatives, like water, plus health education significantly reduce sugared-sweetened beverage consumption in children aged 8 to 18 years.[45] However, improvements are not sustained over time. A meta-analysis reported that school-based behavioral interventions resulted in reductions in sugar-sweetened beverage intake, but the changes were modest.[46] A student-designed and student-led intervention called Sodabriety was piloted with adolescents aged 12 to 18 years in 2 Ohio high schools.[47] The 30-day challenge intervention involved a promotional campaign, facts about soda delivered during daily announcements, and promotion of unsweetened beverages like water, unsweetened tea, and diet soda. Preintervention and postintervention daily sugar-sweetened beverage intake decreased and water intake increased significantly. A school- and community-based water intervention in the Netherlands significantly reduced sugar-sweetened beverage intake for children aged 6 to 12 years (N = 1288).[48] Another systematic review found that home-based interventions are more effective than school-based interventions for children.[49]

One study evaluating state bans on sodas in school vending machines to address pouring rights revealed increased intake of sport drinks, energy drinks, sweetened coffees and teas, and other sugar-sweetened beverages among 9th to 12th grade students, if these other beverages remained available to students.[50] Intake of nonsoda sugar-sweetened beverages did not increase if these other beverages were also removed from the school. This study highlighted the possibility of unhealthy substitution effects associated with soda bans in schools.

To evaluate the effects of warning labels, an online randomized trial involved a hypothetical vending machine task with adolescents aged 12 to 18 years (N = 2202). Participants who received beverages with 1 of 3 safety warning labels significantly reduced hypothetical purchase of sugar-sweetened beverages compared with participants who received beverages with no warning label.[51] The warning label for which there was no significant difference included the words *obesity* rather than *weight gain* and *diabetes* rather than *type 2 diabetes* as noted consequences of drinking sugary beverages.

Sugar-sweetened beverage taxes have significantly reduced per capita intake of sugary beverages in places like New York City,[52] Berkeley, California,[53] Mexico,[54] and Brazil.[55] At least one study from Chile reported modest beverage intake changes associated with sugar-sweetened beverage taxes.[56]

Clinical Strategies to Address Excess Added Sugar Intake

Evidence-based clinical strategies to address added sugar intake have yet to be developed and refined. In the meantime, the following strategies can be used by dental health professionals to address added sugar intake in children.

Collect and record added sugar intake. A routine caries risk assessment should include data collection on the source, amount, and frequency of added sugars consumed by the child.[57] These data should be collected using standardized questions administered at each dental recall visit. Responses should be recorded in the patients' chart and reviewed at subsequent visits to track trends.

Deliver health education consistent with professional guidelines. Sugar-sweetened beverages are one of the main sources of added sugars in children.[58] Parent preferences for sugar-sweetened beverages and availability are strong predictors of child preferences and intake. Dental professionals should provide education regarding 100% fruit juices that is consistent with the American Academy of Pediatric's guidelines.[59] Children younger than 1 year should not be given any fruit juice unless indicated by a health professional. Daily intake should be limited to 4 oz per day for children aged 1 to 3 years, 4 to 6 oz per day for children aged 4 to 6 years, and no more than 8 oz per day (1 cup) for children aged 7 years and older. Furthermore, the American Heart Association recommends that children consume no more than 25 g of sugar per day or 6 teaspoons from all dietary sources.[9] This recommendation means that ideally children should not consume any sugar-sweetened beverages. Plain water and milk are the healthiest beverages. However, restricting sugary beverages for children who are used to sweet drinks or encouraging water intake may not be feasible or effective long-term strategies. For children who demand sugary beverages, sugar-free alternatives are an option. Currently, there is no evidence that sugar-free sweeteners are unsafe for children when consumed in small amounts. Sugar-free sweeteners like sucralose (eg, Splenda) and acesulfame-potassium (eg, Sunett, Sweet One) are well established as safe, based on extensive toxicologic safety data submitted to the US Food and Drug Administration and other regulatory agencies worldwide.[60–64]

Particularly when weighed against the known adverse consequences associated with extreme added sugar intake, including tooth decay and other systemic diseases, the potential benefits of sugar-free beverages outweigh the risks.

Assess readiness to change. Before an attempt is made to help change problematic added sugar behaviors, the caregiver's and/or child's readiness to change should be assessed. The Transtheoretical Model (TTM) posits that there are 5 stages of an individual's readiness to change: precontemplation, contemplation, preparation, action, and maintenance.[65] Attempts at behavior change for individuals in the precontemplation stage may need to be delayed until there is sufficient self-motivation and social support in place to facilitate behavior change. Research on the TTM and dietary change has identified additional processes that facilitate movement between the stages that could help interested individuals engage in healthier behaviors.[66]

Use behavioral methods to supplement health education. Research has shown that health education alone is insufficient in changing health behaviors.[67] Attempts to change patient behaviors should be based on health behavior theories.[68,69] For instance, interventions incorporating concepts from motivational interviewing may help clinicians work with patients to set and monitor health behavior goals.[70] Studies on motivational interviewing in dentistry have yielded mixed results,[71] but other specialties within pediatric medicine have reported success with motivational interviewing-based approaches.[72–74] Other relevant behavioral approaches have been documented, including the application of the Theory of Planned Behavior, which focuses on modifying an individual's intention to take action.[27,74]

Rely on nondental health colleagues. For patients who cannot be managed in a dental setting, dental professionals should work with nutritionists to help patients address excess added sugar intake.[75] The Screening, Brief Intervention, and Referral for Treatment model can be used to systematically refer patients who require specialty care in addressing added sugar intake.[76]

Promote preventive oral health behaviors. For children at increased risk for dental caries, especially for whom added sugar intake is a significant risk factor, dental professionals should reinforce the importance of fluorides. Fluoridated water, toothbrushing with fluoridated toothpaste, and professional fluoride varnish treatments should be recommended. Particular attention should be given to identify caregivers who refuse fluoride, especially among caregivers with children at high-caries risk.[77,78]

Challenges, Opportunities, and Next Steps

The following section outlines current challenges of addressing added sugar intake in children. The goal is to highlight opportunities and provide recommendations on future steps.

There is a dearth of theory-driven socio-behavioral interventions to address added sugar intake. Interventions in dentistry continue to focus almost exclusively on tooth-level strategies (eg, fluoride varnish treatments, sealants, restorative dental treatment) rather than upstream sociodemographic, behavioral, and social determinants of health behaviors that are the root causes of added sugar intake and dental diseases. Fields outside of dentistry, like psychology, sociology, anthropology, and economics, have developed novel theoretic perspectives that could be used to derive potential solutions in dentistry. Dental researchers should continue working with social and behavioral scientists to develop and test interventions rooted in health behavior theories. When developing and refining interventions, end-users from the target community or patient population should be involved to optimize intervention relevance and feasibility.[79] Given the complex etiology of dietary behaviors, interventions should incorporate behavior change at multiple levels relevant for the target population (eg, home, school, community) and address dental as well as nondental disease outcomes using a common risk factors approach.[80,81] Measurement bias in assessing added sugar intake can be minimized by adopting subjective (eg, 24-hour recalls) as well as objective (eg, biomarkers) measures. Sustainability should be part of the intervention planning process to ensure that effective programs can continue without requiring ongoing external resources.[82] Attention to sustainability can also ensure that such programs are more easily disseminated to new communities and populations.

Public health programs need to focus on the highest-risk children. One of the potential unintended consequences of public health programs is widening disparities,[83] especially when the most vulnerable participants are unable to benefit from the program compared with less vulnerable program enrollees. From a health equity perspective, interventions should focus on child subgroups with disproportionately higher levels of dental disease. For instance, based on the sociodemographic factors associated with added sugar presented earlier, one subgroup that might be logically targeted for an added sugar intervention is white children. However, US data indicate caries rates are significantly higher for nonwhite minority children.[84] Thus, an intervention aimed at reducing added sugar intake should focus on minority children to address the highest need subgroup and reduce oral health disparities. There is current intervention work in Alaska Native communities to address sugared fruit drinks and unhealthy foods using community-based approaches appropriate for local populations.[85,86] Both interventions focus on dietary behavior change, though at least one will include caries prevention as an outcome measure.

Local beverage taxes are effective and are part of the solution. Sugar-sweetened beverage taxes reduce intake and may also prevent chronic diseases like obesity.[87] However, depending on local politics, beverage taxes may not be a feasible solution and, in cases like Chicago's soda tax, are easily repealed.[88,89] Federal legislation prevents point-of-sale taxes on beverages purchased through the Supplemental Nutrition Assistance Program (SNAP), and the beverage industry continues to resist local efforts to pass taxes.[90,91] Federal legislation is needed to counter the influence of the beverage industry.[92] Similar to the passing of cigarette taxes to prevent youth tobacco use, beverage taxes should be viewed as part of a multipronged approach to address sugar-sweetened beverage intake in children.[93]

Current sugar intake benchmarks may not be sufficient in preventing caries. The World Health Organization has set the recommended threshold for sugar intake at 10% of the total energy intake.[94] Based on 2011 to 2012 US NHANES data, sugar comprises 17% of the total energy of US children.[95] Data from Japan on the longitudinal relationship between sugar intake and caries suggest that sugar intake needs to be less than 3% or at most 5% of the total energy to prevent caries.[96,97] These stringent benchmarks are not likely to be achieved using the current approaches. Rather than being based on what is realistically achievable, dietary benchmarks should be set on meaningful disease prevention outcomes. The hope is that these benchmarks will encourage researchers, clinicians, policymakers, and others to develop collaborative, holistic, and novel approaches in addressing sugar intake.

Corporate industries are motivated by profits and self-interest. The sugar industry has been likened to Big Tobacco.[98] Corporate industries that support the marketing and distribution of sugar products include food and beverage companies, advertising agencies, and grocers. In addition, schools, hospitals, community centers, and other public spaces where child-related activities and business take place have been complicit in perpetuating access to and consumption of sugars. Beverage labels are difficult for consumers to interpret, and studies show that labels on nearly a quarter of foods and beverages marketed to children overestimate or underestimate the product's listed sugar content by 10%.[99,100] Despite laws allowing industries to self-regulate, advertisers routinely target sugary products to children[101,102]; adverse advertising disproportionately targets low-income and minority children.[103] In addition, there are data exposing the sugar industry's role in suppressing science on the adverse effects of sugar,[104,105] funding studies with null results associated with sugar intake,[106] and influencing the research priorities of federal agencies and public policies.[107,108] As a recent example, the role of the alcohol industry's influence on a study funded by the National Institutes of Health has been publicized.[109] Government regulation and oversight are needed to hold industries and corporations accountable for inaccurate product labeling, illegal advertising, and unethical influence pedaling.[110] To educate the public on the risks associated with sugar, positive and negative front-of-pack labels should be added to sugar-sweetened beverages and public health awareness campaigns should be promulgated.[111,112] Efforts to address pouring rights in schools should ensure that sodas as well as all other sugary beverages are removed from vending machines to avoid substitution effects.[50]

Out-of-date government nutrition programs continue to subsidize the consumption of unhealthy foods and beverages among vulnerable populations. The US Supplemental Nutrition Assistance Program (SNAP) allows sugar-sweetened beverage purchases; the WIC program's allowable food list includes 100% fruit juices, which convey to caregivers that these beverages are healthy. Legislation is required to restrict SNAP purchases, but political and logistic complexities make such legislation unlikely in the near future.[113] In addition, ethical concerns have been raised about restricting choice in vulnerable populations.[114] In the meantime, plausible solutions include incentive-based approaches that allow government nutrition program beneficiaries more flexibility in how funds are spent (eg, Electronic Benefits Transfer use at farmer's markets) or subsidies to encourage healthy spending.[115–118]

In conclusion, sugar-sweetened beverages are a major contributor to dental caries in US children. Future intervention research should account for relevant sociodemographic, behavioral, and social determinants of added sugar intake, which will enable the field to develop and refine evidence-based strategies to prevent dental caries. Dental health professionals are in a position to implement clinical strategies that can help to reduce added sugar intake in patients and should advocate for broader policy-based solutions.

REFERENCES

1. Marcenes W, Kassebaum NJ, Bernabé E, et al. Global burden of oral conditions in 1990-2010: a systematic analysis. J Dent Res 2013;92(7):592–7.
2. Kassebaum NJ, Smith AGC, Bernabé E, et al. GBD 2015 Oral Health Collaborators. Global, Regional, and National Prevalence, Incidence, and Disability-Adjusted Life Years for Oral Conditions for 195 Countries, 1990-2015: A Systematic Analysis for the Global Burden of Diseases, Injuries, and Risk Factors. J Dent Res 2017;96(4):380–7.

3. Hojer JA, Maunsbach AB. The Vipeholm dental caries study: purposes and organisation. Acta Odontol Scand 1954;11(3–4):195–206.
4. Gustafsson BE. The Vipeholm dental caries study: survey of the literature on carbohydrates and dental caries. Acta Odontol Scand 1954;11(3–4):207–31.
5. Gustafsson BE, Quensel C, Swenander Lanke L, et al. The Vipeholm dental caries study; the effect of different levels of carbohydrate intake on caries activity in 436 individuals observed for five years. Acta Odontol Scand 1954;11(3–4): 232–64.
6. Krasse B. The Vipeholm dental caries study: recollections and reflections 50 years later. J Dent Res 2001;80(9):1785–8.
7. World Health Organization (WHO). Guideline: sugars intake for adults and children. 2015. Available at: http://apps.who.int/iris/handle/10665/149782. Accessed August 31, 2018.
8. Fidler Mis N, Braegger C, Bronsky J, et al. ESPGHAN Committee on Nutrition. Sugar in infants, children and adolescents: a position paper of the European Society for Paediatric Gastroenterology, Hepatology and Nutrition Committee on Nutrition. J Pediatr Gastroenterol Nutr 2017;65(6):681–96.
9. Vos MB, Kaar JL, Welsh JA, et al, American Heart Association Nutrition Committee of the Council on Lifestyle and Cardiometabolic Health; council on clinical cardiology; council on cardiovascular disease in the young; council on cardiovascular and stroke nursing; council on epidemiology and prevention; council on functional genomics and translational biology; and council on hypertension. Added sugars and cardiovascular disease risk in children: a scientific statement from the American Heart Association. Circulation 2017;135(19):e1017–34.
10. Marshall TA. Nomenclature, characteristics, and dietary intakes of sugars. J Am Dent Assoc 2015;146(1):61–4.
11. Al Rawahi SH, Asimakopoulou K, Newton JT. Theory based interventions for caries related sugar intake in adults: systematic review. BMC Psychol 2017; 5(1):25.
12. Touger-Decker R, van Loveren C. Sugars and dental caries. Am J Clin Nutr 2003;78(4):881S–92S.
13. Sorensen G, Emmons K, Hunt MK, et al. Model for incorporating social context in health behavior interventions: applications for cancer prevention for working-class, multiethnic populations. Prev Med 2003;37(3):188–97.
14. Eicher-Miller HA, Zhao Y. Evidence for the age-specific relationship of food insecurity and key dietary outcomes among US children and adolescents. Nutr Res Rev 2018;31(1):98–113.
15. Kong A, Odoms-Young AM, Schiffer LA, et al. Racial/ethnic differences in dietary intake among WIC families prior to food package revisions. J Nutr Educ Behav 2013;45(1):39–46.
16. LaRowe TL, Adams AK, Jobe JB, et al. Dietary intakes and physical activity among preschool-aged children living in rural American Indian communities before a family-based healthy lifestyle intervention. J Am Diet Assoc 2010; 110(7):1049–57.
17. Chi DL, Hopkins S, O'Brien D, et al. Association between added sugar intake and dental caries in Yup'ik children using a novel hair biomarker. BMC Oral Health 2015;15(1):121.
18. Drewnowski A, Rehm CD. Consumption of added sugars among US children and adults by food purchase location and food source. Am J Clin Nutr 2014; 100(3):901–7.

19. Bailey RL, Fulgoni VL, Cowan AE, et al. Sources of added sugars in young children, adolescents, and adults with low and high intakes of added sugars. Nutrients 2018;10(1) [pii:E102].

20. Rosinger A, Herrick K, Gahche J, et al. Sugar-sweetened beverage consumption among U.S. youth, 2011-2014. NCHS Data Brief 2017;(271):1–8.

21. Munsell CR, Harris JL, Sarda V, et al. Parents' beliefs about the healthfulness of sugary drink options: opportunities to address misperceptions. Public Health Nutr 2016;19(1):46–54.

22. Pettigrew S, Jongenelis M, Chapman K, et al. Factors influencing the frequency of children's consumption of soft drinks. Appetite 2015;91:393–8.

23. Tipton JA. Caregivers' psychosocial factors underlying sugar-sweetened beverage intake among non-Hispanic black preschoolers: an elicitation study. J Pediatr Nurs 2014;29(1):47–57.

24. Mazarello Paes V, Hesketh K, O'Malley C, et al. Determinants of sugar-sweetened beverage consumption in young children: a systematic review. Obes Rev 2015;16(11):903–13.

25. Harris TS, Ramsey M. Paternal modeling, household availability, and paternal intake as predictors of fruit, vegetable, and sweetened beverage consumption among African American children. Appetite 2015;85:171–7.

26. McClain AD, Chappuis C, Nguyen-Rodriguez ST, et al. Psychosocial correlates of eating behavior in children and adolescents: a review. Int J Behav Nutr Phys Act 2009;6:54.

27. Riebl SK, MacDougal C, Hill C, et al. Beverage choices of adolescents and their parents using the theory of planned behavior: a mixed methods analysis. J Acad Nutr Diet 2016;116(2):226–39.e1.

28. Ezendam NP, Evans AE, Stigler MH, et al. Cognitive and home environmental predictors of change in sugar-sweetened beverage consumption among adolescents. Br J Nutr 2010;103(5):768–74.

29. Beets MW, Tilley F, Kyryliuk R, et al. Children select unhealthy choices when given a choice among snack offerings. J Acad Nutr Diet 2014;114(9):1440–6.

30. Jansen E, Mulkens S, Emond Y, et al. From the Garden of Eden to the land of plenty. Restriction of fruit and sweets intake leads to increased fruit and sweets consumption in children. Appetite 2008;51(3):570–5.

31. Rossen LM, Kobernik EK. Food insecurity and dietary intake among US youth, 2007-2010. Pediatr Obes 2016;11(3):187–93.

32. Tomayko EJ, Mosso KL, Cronin KA, et al. Household food insecurity and dietary patterns in rural and urban American Indian families with young children. BMC Public Health 2017;17(1):611.

33. Sharkey JR, Nalty C, Johnson CM, et al. Children's very low food security is associated with increased dietary intakes in energy, fat, and added sugar among Mexican-origin children (6-11 y) in Texas border Colonias. BMC Pediatr 2012;12:16.

34. Comeau J, Boyle MH. Patterns of poverty exposure and children's trajectories of externalizing and internalizing behaviors. SSM Popul Health 2017;4:86–94.

35. Luff GM, Gray JJ. Complex messages regarding a thin ideal appearing in teenage girls' magazines from 1956 to 2005. Body Image 2009;6(2):133–6.

36. Jansen EC, Miller AL, Lumeng JC, et al. Externalizing behavior is prospectively associated with intake of added sugar and sodium among low socioeconomic status preschoolers in a sex-specific manner. Int J Behav Nutr Phys Act 2017;14(1):135.

37. Santiago-Torres M, Adams AK, Carrel AL, et al. Home food availability, parental dietary intake, and familial eating habits influence the diet quality of urban Hispanic children. Child Obes 2014;10(5):408–15.
38. Ritchie LD, Raman A, Sharma S, et al. Dietary intakes of urban, high body mass index, African American children: family and child dietary attributes predict child intakes. J Nutr Educ Behav 2011;43(4):236–43.
39. Jackson JA, Smit E, Manore MM, et al. The family-home nutrition environment and dietary intake in rural children. Nutrients 2015;7(12):9707–20.
40. Poti JM, Slining MM, Popkin BM. Where are kids getting their empty calories? Stores, schools, and fast-food restaurants each played an important role in empty calorie intake among US children during 2009-2010. J Acad Nutr Diet 2014;114(6):908–17.
41. Dubowitz T, Ghosh-Dastidar M, Cohen DA, et al. Diet and perceptions change with supermarket introduction in a food desert, but not because of supermarket use. Health Aff (Millwood) 2015;34(11):1858–68.
42. Lent MR, Vander Veur S, Mallya G, et al. Corner store purchases made by adults, adolescents and children: items, nutritional characteristics and amount spent. Public Health Nutr 2015;18(9):1706–12.
43. Watts AW, Miller J, Larson NI, et al. Multicontextual correlates of adolescent sugar-sweetened beverage intake. Eat Behav 2018;30:42–8.
44. Bevelander KE, Engels RC, Anschütz DJ, et al. The effect of an intervention on schoolchildren's susceptibility to a peer's candy intake. Eur J Clin Nutr 2013; 67(8):829–35.
45. Avery A, Bostock L, McCullough F. A systematic review investigating interventions that can help reduce consumption of sugar-sweetened beverages in children leading to changes in body fatness. J Hum Nutr Diet 2015;28(Suppl 1): 52–64.
46. Abdel Rahman A, Jomaa L, Kahale LA, et al. Effectiveness of behavioral interventions to reduce the intake of sugar-sweetened beverages in children and adolescents: a systematic review and meta-analysis. Nutr Rev 2018;76(2):88–107.
47. Smith LH, Holloman C. Piloting "sodabriety": a school-based intervention to impact sugar-sweetened beverage consumption in rural Appalachian high schools. J Sch Health 2014;84(3):177–84.
48. van de Gaar VM, Jansen W, van Grieken A, et al. Effects of an intervention aimed at reducing the intake of sugar-sweetened beverages in primary school children: a controlled trial. Int J Behav Nutr Phys Act 2014;11:98.
49. Vargas-Garcia EJ, Evans CEL, Prestwich A, et al. Interventions to reduce consumption of sugar-sweetened beverages or increase water intake: evidence from a systematic review and meta-analysis. Obes Rev 2017;18(11):1350–63.
50. Taber DR, Chriqui JF, Vuillaume R, et al. The association between state bans on soda only and adolescent substitution with other sugar-sweetened beverages: a cross-sectional study. Int J Behav Nutr Phys Act 2015;12(Suppl 1):S7.
51. VanEpps EM, Roberto CA. The influence of sugar-sweetened beverage warnings: a randomized trial of adolescents' choices and beliefs. Am J Prev Med 2016;51(5):664–72.
52. Kansagra SM, Kennelly MO, Nonas CA, et al. Reducing sugary drink consumption: New York City's approach. Am J Public Health 2015;105(4):e61–4.
53. Silver LD, Ng SW, Ryan-Ibarra S, et al. Changes in prices, sales, consumer spending, and beverage consumption one year after a tax on sugar-sweetened beverages in Berkeley, California, US: a before-and-after study. PLoS Med 2017;14(4):e1002283.

54. Colchero MA, Guerrero-López CM, Molina M, et al. Beverages sales in Mexico before and after implementation of a sugar sweetened beverage tax. PLoS One 2016;11(9):e0163463.
55. Claro RM, Levy RB, Popkin BM, et al. Sugar-sweetened beverage taxes in Brazil. Am J Public Health 2012;102(1):178–83.
56. Caro JC, Corvalán C, Reyes M, et al. Chile's 2014 sugar-sweetened beverage tax and changes in prices and purchases of sugar-sweetened beverages: an observational study in an urban environment. PLoS Med 2018;15(7):e1002597.
57. American Academy of Pediatric Dentistry (AAPD). Caries-risk assessment and management for infants, children, and adolescents. Pediatr Dent 2017;39(6): 197–204.
58. National Academies of Sciences, Engineering, and Medicine (NASEM) Health and Medicine Division, et al. Strategies to limit sugar-sweetened beverage consumption in young children: proceedings of a workshop. National Academies Press; 2017.
59. Heyman MB, Abrams SA, Section on Gastroenterology, Hepatology, and Nutrition, Committee on Nutrition. Fruit juice in infants, children, and adolescents: current recommendations. Pediatrics 2017;139(6).
60. Panel on Macronutrients, Panel on the definition of dietary fiber, subcommittee on upper reference levels of nutrients, subcommittee on interpretation and uses of dietary reference intakes, and the standing committee on the scientific evaluation of dietary reference intakes, Institute of Medicine (IOM). Dietary reference intakes for energy, carbohydrate, fiber, fat, fatty acids, cholesterol, protein, and amino acids. National Academies Press; 2005.
61. Magnuson BA, Carakostas MC, Moore NH, et al. Biological fate of low-calorie sweeteners. Nutr Rev 2016;74(11):670–89.
62. Magnuson BA, Roberts A, Nestmann ER. Critical review of the current literature on the safety of sucralose. Food Chem Toxicol 2017;106(Pt A):324–55.
63. Sylvetsky AC, Rother KI. Nonnutritive sweeteners in weight management and chronic disease: a review. Obesity (Silver Spring) 2018;26(4):635–40.
64. Prochaska JO, Redding CA, Evers KE. In: Glanz K, Rimer BK, Viswanath K, editors. In health behavior and health education: theory, research, and practice. 4th edition. John Wiley & Sons; 2008. p. 97–122.
65. Horwath CC, Schembre SM, Motl RW, et al. Does the transtheoretical model of behavior change provide a useful basis for interventions to promote fruit and vegetable consumption? Am J Health Promot 2013;27(6):351–7.
66. Ferris FD, von Gunten CF, Emanuel LL. Knowledge: insufficient for change. J Palliat Med 2001;4(2):145–7.
67. Bartholomew LK, Mullen PD. Five roles for using theory and evidence in the design and testing of behavior change interventions. J Public Health Dent 2011;71(Suppl 1):S20–33.
68. Chi DL. Injecting theory into the dental behavior intervention research process. J Public Health Dent 2011;71(Suppl 1):S35.
69. Ige TJ, DeLeon P, Nabors L. Motivational interviewing in an obesity prevention program for children. Health Promot Pract 2017;18(2):263–74.
70. Chi DL. Motivational interviewing-based approaches in dental practice settings may improve oral health behaviors and outcomes. J Evid Based Dent Pract 2017;17(4):420–1.
71. Nansel TR, Laffel LM, Haynie DL, et al. Improving dietary quality in youth with type 1 diabetes: randomized clinical trial of a family-based behavioral intervention. Int J Behav Nutr Phys Act 2015;12:58.

72. Mallonee LF, Boyd LD, Stegeman C. A scoping review of skills and tools oral health professionals need to engage children and parents in dietary changes to prevent childhood obesity and consumption of sugar-sweetened beverages. J Public Health Dent 2017;77(Suppl 1):S128–35.

73. Dooley D, Moultrie NM, Sites E, et al. Primary care interventions to reduce childhood obesity and sugar-sweetened beverage consumption: Food for thought for oral health professionals. J Public Health Dent 2017;77(Suppl 1):S104–27.

74. Zoellner J, Estabrooks PA, Davy BM, et al. Exploring the theory of planned behavior to explain sugar-sweetened beverage consumption. J Nutr Educ Behav 2012;44(2):172–7.

75. Touger-Decker R, Mobley C, Academy of Nutrition and Dietetics. Position of the academy of nutrition and dietetics: oral health and nutrition. J Acad Nutr Diet 2013;113(5):693–701.

76. Cuevas J, Chi DL. SBIRT-based interventions to improve pediatric oral health behaviors and outcomes: considerations for future behavioral SBIRT interventions in dentistry. Curr Oral Health Rep 2016;3(3):187–92.

77. Chi DL. Parent refusal of topical fluoride for their children: clinical strategies and future research priorities to improve evidence-based pediatric dental practice. Dent Clin North Am 2017;61(3):607–17.

78. Chi DL, Basson A. Surveying dentists' perceptions of caregiver refusal of topical fluoride. JDR Clin Trans Res 2018;3:314–20.

79. D'Alonzo KT. Getting started in CBPR: lessons in building community partnerships for new researchers. Nurs Inq 2010;17(4):282–8.

80. Chi DL. Reducing Alaska Native paediatric oral health disparities: a systematic review of oral health interventions and a case study on multilevel strategies to reduce sugar-sweetened beverage intake. Int J Circumpolar Health 2013;72:21066.

81. Chi DL, Luu M, Chu F. A scoping review of epidemiologic risk factors for pediatric obesity: Implications for future childhood obesity and dental caries prevention research. J Public Health Dent 2017;77(Suppl 1):S8–31.

82. Scheirer MA. Linking sustainability research to intervention types. Am J Public Health 2013;103(4):e73–80.

83. Raittio E, Aromaa A, Kiiskinen U, et al. Income-related inequality in perceived oral health among adult Finns before and after a major dental subsidization reform. Acta Odontol Scand 2016;74(5):348–54.

84. Herzog K, Scott J, Chi DL. Children's oral health inequalities: intersectionality of race, ethnicity, and income. In: Treadwell HM, Evans CA, editors. Oral health in America: removing the stain of disparity. Washington, DC: American Public Health Association; 2019.

85. U.S. Department of Health and Human Services (USDHHS). National Institutes of Health (NIH) Reporter. NIH research portfolio online reporting tools. Project information grant number 1R56DE025813-01A1. 2018a. Reducing sugared fruit drinks in Alaska Native children. Available at: https://projectreporter.nih.gov/. Accessed July 15, 2018.

86. U.S. Department of Health and Human Services (USDHHS). National Institutes of Health (NIH) Reporter. NIH research portfolio online reporting tools. Project information grant number 1R01NR015417-01A1. 2018b. Back to basics: addressing childhood obesity through traditional foods in Alaska. Available at: https://projectreporter.nih.gov/. Accessed July 15, 2018.

87. Cabrera Escobar MA, Veerman JL, Tollman SM, et al. Evidence that a tax on sugar sweetened beverages reduces the obesity rate: a meta-analysis. BMC Public Health 2013;13:1072.

88. KYUK Archives. Talk line. 2013 program. Available at: http://archive.kyuk.org/talk-line-listen-here-to-jan-11-program/. Accessed July 15, 2018.

89. Dewey C. Washington post. Why Chicago's soda tax fizzled after two months — and what it means for the anti-soda movement. 2017. Available at: https://www.washingtonpost.com/news/wonk/wp/2017/10/10/why-chicagos-soda-tax-fizzled-after-two-months-and-what-it-means-for-the-anti-soda-movement/?noredirect=on&utm_term=.dfa5fab81244. Accessed July 15, 2018.

90. Du M, Tugendhaft A, Erzse A, et al. Sugar-sweetened beverage taxes: industry response and tactics. Yale J Biol Med 2018;91(2):185–90.

91. Pomeranz JL. Implications of the supplemental nutrition assistance program tax exemption on sugar-sweetened beverage taxes. Am J Public Health 2015; 105(11):2191–3.

92. Leung CW, Blumenthal SJ, Hoffnagle EE, et al. Associations of food stamp participation with dietary quality and obesity in children. Pediatrics 2013; 131(3):463–72.

93. Lewit EM, Hyland A, Kerrebrock N, et al. Price, public policy, and smoking in young people. Tob Control 1997;6(Suppl 2):S17–24.

94. Moynihan P. Sugars and dental caries: evidence for setting a recommended threshold for intake. Adv Nutr 2016;7(1):149–56.

95. Powell ES, Smith-Taillie LP, Popkin BM. Added sugars intake across the distribution of US children and adult consumers: 1977-2012. J Acad Nutr Diet 2016; 116(10):1543–50.

96. Sheiham A, James WP. A reappraisal of the quantitative relationship between sugar intake and dental caries: the need for new criteria for developing goals for sugar intake. BMC Public Health 2014;14:863.

97. Sheiham A, James WP. A new understanding of the relationship between sugars, dental caries and fluoride use: implications for limits on sugars consumption. Public Health Nutr 2014;17(10):2176–84.

98. Taubes G. The case against sugar. Knopf Doubleday Publishing Group; 2016.

99. Vanderlee L, Goodman S, Sae Yang W, et al. Consumer understanding of calorie amounts and serving size: implications for nutritional labelling. Can J Public Health 2012;103(5):e327–31.

100. Walker RW, Goran MI. Laboratory determined sugar content and composition of commercial infant formulas, baby foods and common grocery items targeted to children. Nutrients 2015;7(7):5850–67.

101. Powell LM, Schermbeck RM, Chaloupka FJ. Nutritional content of food and beverage products in television advertisements seen on children's programming. Child Obes 2013;9(6):524–31.

102. Hingle MD, Castonguay JS, Ambuel DA, et al. Alignment of children's food advertising with proposed federal guidelines. Am J Prev Med 2015;48(6): 707–13.

103. Powell LM, Wada R, Kumanyika SK. Racial/ethnic and income disparities in child and adolescent exposure to food and beverage television ads across the U.S. media markets. Health Place 2014;29:124–31.

104. Kearns CE, Schmidt LA, Glantz SA. Sugar industry and coronary heart disease research: a historical analysis of internal industry documents. JAMA Intern Med 2016;176(11):1680–5.

105. Kearns CE, Apollonio D, Glantz SA. Sugar industry sponsorship of germ-free rodent studies linking sucrose to hyperlipidemia and cancer: an historical analysis of internal documents. PLoS Biol 2017;15(11):e2003460.

106. Litman EA, Gortmaker SL, Ebbeling CB, et al. Source of bias in sugar-sweetened beverage research: a systematic review. Public Health Nutr 2018; 21(12):2345–50.

107. Kearns CE, Glantz SA, Schmidt LA. Sugar industry influence on the scientific agenda of the National Institute of Dental Research's 1971 National Caries Program: a historical analysis of internal documents. PLoS Med 2015;12(3): e1001798.

108. Kearns C, Schmidt L, Apollonio D, et al. The sugar industry's influence on policy. Science 2018;360(6388):501.

109. Wadman M. NIH pulls the plug on controversial alcohol trial. Science magazine. 2018. Available at: http://www.sciencemag.org/news/2018/06/nih-pulls-plug-controversial-alcohol-trial. Accessed July 15, 2018.

110. Popkin BM, Hawkes C. Sweetening of the global diet, particularly beverages: patterns, trends, and policy responses. Lancet Diabetes Endocrinol 2016; 4(2):174–86.

111. Pomeranz JL, Mozaffarian D, Micha R. Can the government require health warnings on sugar-sweetened beverage advertisements? JAMA 2018;319(3):227–8.

112. Boles M, Adams A, Gredler A, et al. Ability of a mass media campaign to influence knowledge, attitudes, and behaviors about sugary drinks and obesity. Prev Med 2014;67(Suppl 1):S40–5.

113. U.S. Department of Agriculture (USDA). Food and nutrition service. Implications of restriction the use of food stamp benefits. 2007. Available at: http://fns-prod. azureedge.net/sites/default/files/FSPFoodRestrictions.pdf. Accessed July 1, 2018.

114. Chrisinger BW. Ethical imperatives against item restriction in the Supplemental Nutrition Assistance Program. Prev Med 2017;100:56–60.

115. Robles B, Montes CE, Nobari TZ, et al. Dietary behaviors among public health center clients with electronic benefit transfer access at farmers' markets. J Acad Nutr Diet 2017;117(1):58–68.

116. Richards MR, Sindelar JL. Rewarding healthy food choices in SNAP: behavioral economic applications. Milbank Q 2013;91(2):395–412.

117. Ammerman AS, Hartman T, DeMarco MM. Behavioral economics and the supplemental nutrition assistance program: making the healthy choice the easy choice. Am J Prev Med 2017;52(2S2):S145–50.

118. Epstein LH, Finkelstein E, Raynor H, et al. Experimental analysis of the effect of taxes and subsides on calories purchased in an on-line supermarket. Appetite 2015;95:245–51.

Analgesic Therapy in Dentistry
From a Letter to the Editor to an Evidence-Base Review

Paul A. Moore, DMD, PhD, MPH[a],*, Elliot V. Hersh, DMD, MS, PhD[b]

KEYWORDS

- Evidence-based therapy • Analgesics • Acute pain • Third-molar extractions
- Opioid-sparing pain management

KEY POINTS

- Historically, recommendations for pain management relied on practitioner experience, with little valid clinical research available.
- The era of randomized placebo-controlled clinical trials using third-molar extraction surgery greatly expanded our understanding of analgesic efficacy and safety.
- Meta-analyses of data from more than 460 clinical analgesic trials allow clinicians to compare the benefits and harms associated with analgesics used for acute pain.

North America is facing an escalating opioid addiction crisis that was created to a great extent by inappropriate prescribing of opioid analgesics for the management of pain. During the 1990s, various advocacy groups lobbied the medical community to improve chronic pain management in the United States. These patient groups estimated that millions of people were unnecessarily suffering because of failed or inadequate treatment of their chronic pain. The medical community responded, with support of The Joint Commission, by establishing pain as the "fifth" vital sign and recommended that all patients, as part of routine evaluation, should, in addition to recording blood pressure, pulse, respiratory rate, and body temperature, be queried regarding possible pain symptoms. It was thought that identifying and prioritizing patients' pain symptoms would promote better chronic pain management.

Disclosure Statement: See last page of the article.
[a] Pharmacology, Dental Public Health, University of Pittsburgh School of Dental Medicine, 386 Salk Hall, Pittsburgh, PA 15261, USA; [b] Department of Oral Surgery and Pharmacology, University of Pennsylvania School of Dental Medicine, 240 South 40th Street, Philadelphia, PA 19104-6030, USA
* Corresponding author.
E-mail address: pam7@pitt.edu

Dent Clin N Am 63 (2019) 35–44
https://doi.org/10.1016/j.cden.2018.08.004
0011-8532/19/© 2018 Elsevier Inc. All rights reserved.

Unfortunately, recognizing patients' pain condition without the availability of evidence-based treatments did not necessarily translate into better treatment.

As a strategy to better manage chronic pain, the medical community began using more opioid analgesics, particularly delayed-release formulations, to provide pain relief. Opioid prescribing increased tenfold during the period of 2000 to 2016. This dramatic increase in prescription opioids resulted in an increase in the availability and subsequent misuse of these addictive pain medications. This misuse and abuse of opioid analgesics has been shown to be closely correlated with increased emergency department visits for overdose reactions.

It has been known for centuries that opioids are highly addictive when consumed for prolonged periods of time. Pharmacologic tolerance to the efficacy of opioid analgesic results in a need for increased dosing. The more recently described phenomena of opioid-induced hyperalgesia whereby some patients actually become more sensitive to pain-provoking stimuli further adds to the quandary. One must question the source of evidence that justified the belief that prescription opioids were safe and effective for treating chronic pain.

Pain management has historically relied on clinical experience that emphasizes the "art" component of the accepted "art-and-science" approach to medicine. Essentially only 3 drugs were considered effective pain relievers before 1970: aspirin (ASA), acetaminophen (APAP), and agents derived from opium (eg, morphine, codeine). Selection of an agent and determination of proper doses were empirical and relied on clinical knowledge and the accepted principles of "in-my-hands" recommendations. Formal scientific assessments of efficacy and safety were uncommon; placebo-controlled studies were rare; analgesic therapies focused mainly on hospitalized patients with cancer pain, headache, and postsurgical pain, such as episiotomy. Well-established clinical evidence for analgesic efficacy and safety was lacking.

A LETTER TO THE EDITOR IN THE *NEW ENGLAND JOURNAL OF MEDICINE*: 1980

Long-acting opioids, such as Oxycontin®, one of the most notoriously abused delayed-release opioids ever marketed, were promoted as safe treatments for managing chronic non-cancer pain by their pharmaceutical manufacturers. With little clinical evidence, delayed-released opioids were presented to the medical community as being able to establish relatively constant blood levels, so that cravings for re-administration, that may be associated with rapid drug elimination and rapid lowering of opioid blood levels, would not occur. The dangers of opioid drug dependence were downplayed, in part, by relying on scant evidence such as the letter to the editor of the *New England Journal of Medicine* published in 1980. This short, 101-word letter sent by Jane Porter and Hershel Jick of the Boston Collaborative Drug Surveillance Program was misrepresented to imply that addiction and dependence associated with opioid analgesics was rare (4 patients of 11,882 hospital patients examined).[1]

The letter is available in its entirety from the *New England Journal of Medicine*.[1] It has been reproduced on several websites,[2–5] a book entitled *Dreamland* by Sam Quinones describing the development of the current opioid crisis,[6] and most recently in a thoughtful letter in the *New England Journal of Medicine* that critically addressed the 608 citations and the overall misuse of Porter and Jick's observation within the medical community.[7] See https://www.nejm.org/doi/10.1056/NEJM198001103020221.

This brief "letter to the editor" was written to provide a rapid unstructured observation of the narcotic addiction potential when immediate-acting opioids are administered in a physician controlled and monitored hospital environment, provided for treatment of acute pain, and given to patients with no history of drug addiction. It was never intended to be a scientific study. It was never intended to describe addiction risk associated with unsupervised administration outside of a hospital environment. It was never able to suggest addiction potential with chronic administration.

Elements of the 101-word letter included:

1. The 11,882 patients included were all "hospitalized medical patients."
   "...we examined our current files to determine the incidence of narcotic addiction in 39,946 hospitalized medical patients' who were monitored consecutively."[1]
2. Patient demographics, selection criteria, or opioid regimen are not provided.
   "...there were 11,882 patients who received at least one narcotic preparation."[1]
3. Definitions and diagnoses of "addiction" or "history of addiction" were not stated.
   "...there were only four cases of reasonably well documented addiction in patients who had a history of addiction."[1]
4. The concluding sentence makes it clear that the abstract was not describing long term administration of opioids for treating chronic pain in an unsupervised outpatient setting.
   "....despite widespread use of narcotic drugs in hospitals, the development of addiction is rare in medical patients with no history of addiction."[1]
5. As a brief letter, the duration of hospital stay and reason for these medical patients' hospitalization are not provided.

The Boston Collaborative Drug Surveillance Program was a hospital-based program that assessed drug side effects among post-operative and burn inpatients, and had little capability to identify, evaluate and document the addiction potential of long-term outpatient opioid therapy. Clearly the observation had been drastically misinterpreted when considering chronic pain patients. Its impact may have been due to the prestige of the *New England Journal of Medicine* where this letter to the editor was published. Certainly, the importance and relevance of the letter was incorrectly presented as valid evidence for the safe and non-addictive use in treating chronic pain.

Thankfully, the requirements for evidence-based analgesic therapy have changed.

RANDOMIZED PLACEBO-CONTROLLED CLINICAL TRIALS FOR PAIN ASSESSMENT

A major contribution to our knowledge of the safety and efficacy of oral analgesics comes from an outpatient methodology described by Steve Cooper and William Beaver during the 1970s. These clinical pharmacologists developed and validated a method to assess the efficacy of analgesics for pain relief following the common outpatient dental procedure of third-molar (wisdom tooth) extraction. The postoperative pain model demonstrated sensitivity in distinguishing oral analgesic medications from placebos and other active drugs.[8] The availability of such a large potential population requiring acute postoperative pain management facilitated the utility of this clinical pain model.

The power of the model for collecting clinical trial data regarding analgesic safety and efficacy was based on its straightforward categories for recording pain intensity and pain relief, the reasonably homogeneous nature of the surgical trauma of the third-molar extraction procedure, and a large population of young, healthy subjects available for enrollment. It has been estimated that 3.5 million young adults undergo the extraction of their wisdom teeth every year in the United States.[9]

As newer nonsteroidal antiinflammatory drugs (NSAIDs), such as ibuprofen and naproxen, were being developed in the 1970s through the 1990s, this efficient pain assessment model was commonly employed. The model was accepted by the Food and Drug Administration (FDA) to demonstrate the efficacy and safety indications for new analgesic drug applications. This placebo-controlled clinical drug trial model has been used, with some variation and modification, for almost all of the analgesics marketed today in North America.

The clinical pain model enrolls subjects planning to undergo third-molar extractions. To assure adequate surgical trauma, most clinical trials require at least one of the teeth to be impacted within the lower jaw bone (mandible). This outpatient surgical procedure requires local anesthesia and often an intravenous sedation regimen and is completed for all enrolled subjects. Following surgery, as the local anesthesia wears off and pain intensity reaches a moderate to severe level, subjects are provided one of several blinded treatment options, usually in a parallel design. In addition to a placebo, the research design usually includes a known comparator (ie, acetaminophen) and the medications to be evaluated. A rescue medication is provided if subjects have pain that is not adequately managed by their treatment medication.

Pain is assessed before any of the drug treatments are administered and at hourly intervals. Pain intensity is recorded using categories of severe (3) moderate (2) slight (1) and or none (0). Pain relief is recorded hourly as complete (4) a lot (3) some (2) a little (1) or none (0). The pain intensity measures are transformed into pain intensity difference (PID) from baseline. For example, **Fig 1** illustrates the mean hourly responses of each PID measures over the period of study. Summary statistics for the drugs' overall effectiveness often uses the sum of all hourly PIDs weighted over time [SPIDs] and the sum of hourly pain relief scores weighted over time [TOTPARs].

The third-molar extraction pain model usually reports results as pain intensity, PID, SPID and TOTPAR. Additional measures have been included in this model to determine the point when pain is reduced by 50% of the starting pain (Pain Half-Gone), or pain estimated using Visual Analog Scales (VAS) pain ratings (measured on a line anchored from none to worst pain) have been used. Analgesic onset recorded as time to first perceptible and meaningful relief via stopwatch measures, remedication times when a rescue pain reliever is administered, and Global Satisfaction scores are often included in the study design and data analyses.

Because these data assess inflammatory postoperative pain following oral surgery, the relevance to dentists cannot be understated. It can be clearly seen in **Fig. 1** that the placebo is the least effective pain reliever and that ibuprofen 400 mg is the most

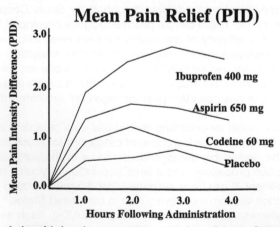

Fig. 1. Example of the third-molar extraction model used in a clinical trial of aspirin, ibuprofen, codeine, and placebo. (*Data from* Cooper SA, Engel J, Ladov M, et al. Analgesic efficacy of a Ibuprofen-codeine combination. Pharmacotherapy 1982;2(3):162–7.)

effective. The results can vary from one study to another because of differences in the patient population's age and severity of the surgical trauma. Often multiple study sites using different research personnel have been used to identify sources of variability and improve the validity of the findings.

QUANTITATIVE SYSTEMATIC REVIEWS OF INDIVIDUAL ANALGESICS

Because of the similarities of the oral surgical procedure, the patient populations, and the outcome pain and pain relief measure used in these clinical trials, multiple published clinical research studies that investigate the same analgesic agent can be combined to preform systematic reviews. Combining data taken from multiple clinical trials data collected for APAP clinical trials using the third-molar model is a good example of this methodology.[10]

This quantitative review summarizes 6 single-dose randomized controlled clinical trials (RCCTs) that evaluated the analgesic efficacy of both a placebo and APAP 500 mg. The 6 studies all met the inclusion criteria and were judged to be of high quality and properly performed. Overall, a total of 561 subjects were included in this meta-analysis: 290 receiving APAP and 271 receiving placebo.[10] The graphic on the right of **Fig. 2**, called a Forrest plot, summarizes and consolidates the findings of studies. The size of the solid square indicates the number of subjects in the individual study. As illustrated, study 5 has a small square representing a total of 90 subjects, whereas study 3 has a larger square representing 206 subjects. The horizontal position of the solid square represents the risk ratio values and indicates how well APAP works as compared with the placebo. For study 1, the ratio is 1.03 indicating that in this study the number of subjects with pain relief is almost identical for APAP and placebo. The overall risk ratio, shown by the solid diamond, is a summary score that is weighted to adjust for the different samples sizes of the individual studies. In this example, the percentage of subjects experiencing at least 50% pain relief following a single dose of APAP 500 mg was 61% (176 of 290). The percentage of

Sample Forrest Plot
Acetaminophen 500 mg vs Placebo

	Acetaminophen		Placebo			Risk Ratio	Risk Ratio
	Events	Total	Events	Total	Weight	Value [95% CI]	Value [95% CI]
Study #1	11	37	11	38	12%	1.03 [0.5, 2.0]	
Study #2	54	72	25	76	28%	2.28 [1.6, 3.2]	
Study #3	46	81	22	57	29%	1.47 [1.01, 2.2]	
Study #4	24	29	10	29	11%	2.40 [1.4, 4.1]	
Study #5	22	30	8	30	9%	2.75 [1.5, 5.2]	
Study #6	19	41	10	41	11%	1.90 [1.01, 3.6]	
Overall	176	290	86	271	100%	1.91 [1.6, 2.3]	

```
        0.2      0.5   1.0   2.0    5.0
        Favors Placebo      Favors Acetaminophen
```

Fig. 2. A sample Forrest plot that illustrates the graphical presentation of 6 clinical trials of the efficacy of APAP 500 mg compared with placebo in providing pain relief following the surgical extraction of third molars. CI, confidence interval. (*Data from* Toms L, McQuay HJ, Derry S, et al. Single dose oral paracetamol (acetaminophen) for postoperative pain in adults. Cochrane Database Syst Rev 2008;(4):CD004602.)

subjects experiencing at least 50% pain relief following a single dose of the placebo was 32% (86 of 271).

By combining the results of several studies, a meta-analysis is able to combine the findings of multiple RCCTs, increase the overall sample size, and create much more confidence in the finding that one treatment is better than another. In this example, the summary value of APAP indicates the overall risk ratio of 1.91 (1.6, 2.3, 95% confidence interval [CI]) indicates that APAP 500 mg is statistically a more effective analgesic than a placebo.

COCHRANE REVIEWS OF MULTIPLE ANALGESIC AGENTS

Some of the most comprehensive evidence-based knowledge of the efficacy of analgesic agents has been correlated and published by the Cochrane Collaborative. Using the results of meta-analyses of individual quantitative reviews (as indicated by the earlier example), the Cochrane Collaborative investigators are able to create a probability statistic that is common to all studies, the number-needed-to-treat (NNT), that can be used to compare all analgesic medications that use the third-molar extraction model. The NNT statistic represents the reciprocal of the absolute risk reduction value based on one of the pain relief outcomes. The outcome of 50% maximum pain relief over the duration of individual studies is often used because it is considered clinically meaningful.

In terms of pain medications, the NNT represents the number of people who must be treated by a specific dose of pain medication to have one person achieve clinically meaningful pain relief. The lower the NNT, the more effective the analgesic. For example, an analgesic with an NNT of 1 means that the analgesic medicine is 100% effective at reducing pain; everyone who takes the medicine has effective pain relief. An analgesic with an NNT of 2 means 2 people must be treated in order for one to receive clinically meaningful relief. For oral pain medications, an NNT of 1.5 would be considered excellent and an NNT of 2.5 would be considered very good, whereas a drug with an NNT of 10 would not be considered an effective analgesic (ie, 10 people would have to be treated for 1 person to experience pain relief).

The data from randomized controlled trials studying single-dose oral analgesics in acute postoperative pain come almost exclusively from studies involving patients who have undergone surgical extraction of their third molars (wisdom teeth). It derives from the analysis of 39 Cochrane reviews by R. Andrew Moore and his colleagues[11] with the Cochrane Collaborative. This overview of meta-analyses includes only high-quality clinical trials that were both randomized and properly blinded. The results were established from nearly 58,000 adult participants of nearly 460 individual clinical trials.[11]

The analgesics commonly prescribed in North America are shown in **Table 1**.[12] Two APAP 500 mg (2 Tylenol Extra Strength tablets) have an NNT of 3.2. Ibuprofen 400 mg (2 Advil tablets), with an NNT of 2.3, is shown to be a more effective analgesic. Surprisingly, oxycodone 10 mg combined with APAP 650 mg (2 Percocet tablets) has a similar NNT as ibuprofen 400 mg of 2.3. The best NNT reported is for the combination ibuprofen 200 mg/APAP 500 mg, which has an NNT 1.6, although it does represent the smallest sample size analyzed.

The methodology to determine the efficacy of a treatment can be extended to include an evaluation of adverse effects of treatment. The expanded NNT statistic is now redefined to determine the number-need-to-treat-to-benefit (NNTB) and number-needed-to-treat-to-harm (NNTH). The utility of this statistic (NNTH) is somewhat compromised because the sample sizes of clinical trials are powered to determine efficacy and may not be large enough to determine a specific side effect. In a review of reviews recently

Table 1		
Relative analgesic efficacy of oral analgesics		
Drug Formulation	**Trials/ Subjects**	**NNT (95% CI)**
Aspirin 600/650 mg	45/3581	4.5 (4.0–5.2)
APAP 1000 mg	19/2157	3.2 (2.9–3.6)
Celecoxib 400 mg	4/620	2.5 (2.2–2.9)
Ibuprofen 400 mg	49/5428	2.3 (2.2–2.4)
Oxycodone 10 mg plus APAP 650 mg	6/673	2.3 (2.0–6.4)
Naproxen 500/550 mg	5/402	1.8 (1.6–2.1)
Ibuprofen 200 mg plus APAP 500 mg	2/280	1.6 (1.4–1.8)

published, an assessment of the NNTH for oral analgesics concluded that opioid combinations were more likely to have side effects, usually nausea/vomiting and dizziness.[13]

Certainly, evidence-based decision-making to evaluate the balance between benefits and harm is limited by the source of data. Adverse drug events reported from acute analgesic studies are limited to reporting methods. Long-term adverse outcomes, such as the potential for drug abuse and addiction, cannot be assessed from short-term single-dose dental pain studies. Although a somewhat more comprehensive understanding of the side effects of a drug can be obtained by 5- to 7-day multidose studies, whereby the first placebo arm is rerandomized into one of the active treatment groups, this design still lacks the sensitivity to establish the abuse potential of a drug.[14]

TRANSLATING EVIDENCE INTO THERAPEUTIC GUIDELINES AND TREATMENT STRATEGIES

Evidence-based knowledge for the efficacy and safety of oral analgesics can be applied toward creating recommendations for treating postoperative pain in dentistry. The findings established and presented by the Cochrane database support the efficacy of NSAIDs and the potential harm associated with the use opioid analgesics. Additionally, understanding the additive analgesia associated with the combination of an NSAID and APAP provides support for the use of this combination as a potential alternative to prescribing analgesics containing opioids. This alternative has been applied toward a step-wise approach to treating dental postoperative pain (**Table 2**).

When recommending the ibuprofen-APAP combination, the specific dose of ibuprofen and APAP should be tailored to patient needs and the practitioner's expectations for postoperative pain. When evaluating ibuprofen alone in impacted third-molar postsurgical dental pain patients, the 400-mg dose seems to provide better analgesia than the 200-mg dose, whereas 600 mg ibuprofen has even better analgesia.[11–13] Thus, in patients with moderate to severe pain, a full therapeutic dose of ibuprofen combined with APAP may be required for achieving the most effective analgesic response.

In considering a pain management strategy that requires NSAIDs, one must be alert to adverse drug reactions as well. NSAIDs, such as ibuprofen and naproxen, should be avoided in many patient populations, such as those with a history of peptic ulcer, stomach bleeding, and uncontrolled hypertension with preexisting renal disease. In addition, patients on anticoagulant or lithium therapy may exhibit a heightened bleeding risk or classic lithium toxicity if NSAIDs are prescribed to these populations.[15]

The FDA has alerted practitioners and consumers of potential liver toxicity associated with excessive dosing with acetaminophen. Acute liver failure caused by

Table 2
Opioid-sparing treatments for acute pain

Pain Severity	Analgesic Recommendation
Mild pain	Ibuprofen 200–400 mg q 4–6 h: as needed for pain
Mild-moderate pain	Ibuprofen 400–600 mg q 6 h: fixed interval for 24 h Then ibuprofen 400 mg q 4–6 h: as needed for pain
Moderate-severe pain	Ibuprofen 400–600 mg plus APAP 500 mg q 6 h: fixed interval for 24 h Then ibuprofen 400 mg plus APAP 500 mg q 6 h: as needed for pain
Severe pain	Ibuprofen 400–600 mg plus APAP 650/hydrocodone 10 mg q 6 h: fixed interval for 24–48 h Then ibuprofen 400–600 mg plus APAP 650 mg q 6 h: as needed for pain

Cautions and considerations: (1) Patients should be cautioned to avoid excessive APAP (greater than 4000 mg/d) and to check to determine if APAP is included in other combination medications. (2) Maximum dosage of ibuprofen is 2400 mg per day. (3) For many patients, NSAIDs are contraindicated. Alternative therapy, including APAP-opioid analgesic, may be an effective alternative.

unintentional consumption of excessive APAP has been reported. Toxicity induced by APAP has been reported when a daily dose of 4000 mg is exceeded.[16] When prescribing APAP for the management of acute postoperative pain, one must be careful to limit the dosing regimen to avoid potential overdose. Patients should be cautioned to follow dosing instructions and avoid the concomitant use of the many other OTC formulations that contain APAP.

Effective alternatives to opioid-containing analgesics may be a strategy to prevent potential prescription drug abuse and diversion, a national concern associated with dispensing opioid prescription drugs. Increasing one's reliance on nonopioid postoperative analgesics should not be the sole opioid-sparing strategy for postoperative pain control. The use of the long-acting local anesthetic of 0.5% bupivacaine with 1:200,000 epinephrine to provide extended soft tissue and periosteal anesthesia has been found to be an effective strategy to limit the need for oral analgesics. The use of the corticosteroid dexamethasone has been demonstrated to be effective in limiting trismus and pain following third-molar surgery. Additionally, the use of a peripherally-acting analgesics, such as ibuprofen or naproxen, before surgery to preemptively manage postoperative sequelae has been found to decrease the severity and onset of acute postoperative pain.[17] All of these strategies have been used by oral surgeons for pain management following third-molar extractions.

SUMMARY

An extremely large database of analgesic efficacy and safety has been created to a great extent because of common research methodologies. This database has allowed investigators to apply evidence-based methodologies to quantify and compare oral analgesics. More recently published findings are changing the strategies for therapy that focus on opioid-sparing pain management alternatives. The demonstrated efficacy of postoperative pain relief using the combination of ibuprofen and APAP provides a potentially valuable strategy for postoperative pain management in dentistry and an alternative to prescription opioid formulations following dental surgery.

DISCLOSURE STATEMENT

In the last 20 years, Dr P.A. Moore has served as a research consultant to several pharmaceutical companies, including Dentsply Pharmaceutical, Kodak Dental

Systems, Septodont USA, St Renatus, Novalar Inc, and Novocol of Canada Inc. His responsibilities have involved research protocol development of new anesthetics used in dentistry as well as pharmacovigilance of marketed local anesthetic products. None of these interactions have an impact on the current article and none are currently active. Over the last 25 years, Dr E.V. Hersh, representing the Trustees of the University of Pennsylvania, has received research grant monies from the following sources: Pfizer Consumer Healthcare, Wyeth Ayerst, AAI Pharmaceuticals, Novocol (Septodont) of Canada, Novalar, Septodont USA, Church and Dwight, St Renatus, Sanofi Pharmaceuticals, Charleston Laboratories, Parke-Davis Pharmaceuticals, Cetylite Inc, the University of Pennsylvania Research Foundation, the PENN Dental Medicine Rabinowitz Endowment, and NIH. He has also been a consultant for Charleston Labs and McNeil Pharmaceuticals. These consulting responsibilities have involved clinical drug development and the construction of expert reports on previously published data.

REFERENCES

1. Porter J, Jick H. Addiction rare in patients treated with narcotics. N Engl J Med 1980;302(2):123.
2. Available at: https://en.wikipedia.org/wiki/Addiction_Rare_in_Patients_Treated_with_Narcotics. Accessed September 30, 2018.
3. Available at: https://www.businessinsider.com/porter-and-jick-letter-launched-the-opioid-epidemic-2016-5. Accessed September 30, 2018.
4. Available at: https://www.researchgate.net/publication/15849526_Addiction_Rare_in_Patients_Treated_with_Narcotics. Accessed September 30, 2018.
5. Available at: http://www.slate.com/articles/health_and_science/science/2017/06/how_bad_footnotes_helped_cause_the_opioid_crisis.html. Accessed September 30, 2018.
6. Quinones S. Dreamland: the true tale of America's Opiate Epidemic. New York: Bloomsbury Press; 2015.
7. Leung PTM, Macdonald EM, Stanbrook MB, et al. A 1980 letter on the risk of opioid addiction. N Engl J Med 2017;376:2194–5.
8. Cooper SA, Beaver WT. A model to evaluate mild analgesics in oral surgery outpatients. Clin Pharmacol Ther 1976;20(2):241–50.
9. Moore PA, Nahouraii HS, Zovko J, et al. Dental therapeutic practice patterns in the U.S. I: anesthesia and sedation. Gen Dent 2006;54(2):92–8.
10. Toms L, McQuay HJ, Derry S, et al. Single dose oral paracetamol (acetaminophen) for postoperative pain in adults. Cochrane Database Syst Rev 2008;(4): CD004602.
11. Moore RA, Derry S, McQuay HJ, et al. Single dose oral analgesics for acute postoperative pain in adults (review). Cochrane Database Syst Rev 2011;(9):CD008659.
12. Moore PA, Hersh EV. Combining Ibuprofen and acetaminophen for acute postoperative pain management: translating clinical research to dental practice. J Am Dent Assoc 2013;144(8):898–908.
13. Moore PA, Ziegler KM, Lipman RD, et al. Benefits and harms associated with analgesic medications used in the management of acute dental pain: an overview of systematic reviews. J Am Dent Assoc 2018;149(4):256–68.
14. Hersh EV, Cooper SA, Betts N, et al. Single dose and multidose analgesic efficacy and safety study of meclofenamate sodium and ibuprofen. Oral Surg Oral Med Oral Pathol 1993;76:680–7.

15. Hersh EV, Moore PA. Three serious drug interactions that every dentist should know about. Compend Contin Educ Dent 2015;36:408–13.
16. Guggenheimer J, Moore PA. Therapeutic applications and risks associated with acetaminophen: a review and update. J Am Dent Assoc 2011;142(12):38–44.
17. Hersh EV, Kane WT, O'Neil M, et al. Prescribing recommendations for the treatment of acute pain in dentistry. Compend Contin Educ Dent 2011;32:22–30.

Evidence-Based Dentistry Update on Silver Diamine Fluoride

Yasmi O. Crystal, DMD, MSc[a],*, Richard Niederman, DMD[b]

KEYWORDS

- Silver diamine fluoride • Dental caries • Caries arrest • Caries management
- Pediatric dentistry

KEY POINTS

- Silver diamine fluoride incorporates the antibacterial effects of silver and the remineralizing actions of a high-concentration fluoride. It effectively arrests the disease process on most lesions treated.
- Systematic reviews of clinical trials confirm the effectiveness of silver diamine fluoride as a caries-arresting agent for primary teeth and root caries and its ease of use, low cost, and relative safety.
- No caries removal is necessary to arrest the caries process, so the use of silver diamine fluoride is appropriate when other forms of caries control are not available or feasible.
- A sign of arrest is the dark staining of the lesions and affected tooth structures. That could be a deterrent for patients who have esthetic concerns. A thorough informed consent is recommended to ensure high patient satisfaction.
- Silver diamine fluoride use for caries control is recommended as part of a comprehensive caries management program, where individual needs and risks are considered.

Disclosure: Research reported in this work was partially funded by the National Institute on Minority Health and Health Disparities of the National Institutes of Health under Awards Numbers R01MD011526 and a Patient-Centered Outcomes Research Institute (PCORI) award (PCS-1609-36824). The views presented in this publication are solely the responsibility of the authors and do not necessarily represent the official views of the National Institutes of Health or the Patient-Centered Outcomes Research Institute (PCORI), its Board of Governors or Methodology Committee.

[a] Pediatric Dentistry, New York University College of Dentistry, 345 East 24th Street. 9W, New York, NY 10010, USA; [b] Department of Epidemiology & Health Promotion, New York University College of Dentistry, 433 1st Avenue, Room 720, New York, NY 10010, USA
* Corresponding author. Department of Pediatric Dentistry, 345 East 24th Street. 9W, New York, NY 10010.
E-mail address: yoc1@nyu.edu

Dent Clin N Am 63 (2019) 45–68
https://doi.org/10.1016/j.cden.2018.08.011
0011-8532/19/© 2018 Elsevier Inc. All rights reserved.

INTRODUCTION

The global burden of oral disease and the negative social and economic effect associated with it, are a growing problem worldwide.[1]

The widespread use of water fluoridation and fluoride-containing oral products produced significant decreases in the prevalence and severity of dental caries over the last 70 years.[2,3] However, the benefits of these prevention interventions have not materialized in all segments of society in most countries. Free sugars and processed carbohydrates as a component of diet have increased in many countries, both developed and developing alike. As Thompson and colleagues[4] have shown, lower income groups are particularly vulnerable to high dietary sugar intake. The result has been a disparity in caries experience across socioeconomic groups. In the United States and other high-income countries, untreated dental decay in children is strongly patterned by income and ethnicity, mainly owing to cost and limited availability and/or access to services.[5] In lower income groups, much of the caries goes untreated, resulting in severe disease levels that leads to pain, expense, and a decreased quality of life for the affected children and their families.[6]

Even when dental services are accessible, traditional restorative treatment can be difficult to deliver to young children with severe disease and those with special management considerations.[7] To address this difficulty, advanced forms of behavior management like sedation and/or general anesthesia are often used, which increase the cost and the risk for the patient and the dentist.[8] Elderly patients often face similar challenges, because increasing rates of untreated decay can severely affect their quality of life, and the difficulties of receiving dental care are accentuated by limitations with mobility and other comorbidities.[9]

When it comes to prevention, epidemiologic studies indicate that when the bacterial challenge is high or the salivary components are lacking, natural remineralization or that aided by fluoride products is insufficient to prevent or arrest the caries process. Thus, there is an urgent need to find ways to beneficially modify the biofilm and to enhance the remineralization process to decrease caries experience and attain improved outcomes of oral health.[10] This situation calls for a paradigm change in caries prevention and management. Specifically, we need more effective, affordable, accessible, and safe treatments that are easy to implement in different settings, and are available to the most vulnerable populations.[11]

Silver diamine fluoride (SDF), a clear liquid that combines the antibacterial effects of silver and the remineralizing effects of fluoride, is a promising therapeutic agent for managing caries lesions in young children and those with special care needs that has only recently become available in the United States. Multiple in vitro studies document its effectiveness in reducing specific cariogenic bacteria[12] and its remineralizing potential on enamel and dentin.[13,14] Its in vivo mechanism(s) of action are a subject of ongoing research. What is currently understood is that the fluoride component strengthens the tooth structure under attack by the acid byproducts of bacterial metabolism,[15] decreasing its solubility, but SDF may also interfere with the biofilm, killing bacteria that cause the local environmental imbalance that demineralizes dental tissues.[16] Thus, SDF becomes one of the tools available to address caries by modifying the bacterial actions on the tissue while enhancing remineralization.

Numerous systematic reviews substantiate SDF's efficacy for caries arrest in primary teeth, and arrest and prevention of new root caries lesions. It meets the US Institute of Medicine's 6 quality aims of being[7]:

1. Safe—clinical trials that have used it in more than 3800 individuals have reported no serious adverse events[7,17];

2. Effective—arrests approximately 80% of treated lesions[18];
3. Efficient—can be applied by health professionals in different health and community settings with minimal preparation in less than 1 minute;
4. Timely—its ease of application can allow its use as an intervention agent as soon as the problem is diagnosed;
5. Patient centered—is minimally invasive and painless, meeting the immediate needs of a child or adult in 1 treatment session; and
6. Equitable—its application is equally effective and affordable; with the medicament costing less than $1 per application, it is a viable treatment for lower income groups.

The only apparent drawback is that as the caries lesions become arrested, the precipitation of silver byproducts in the dental tissues stain the lesions black, which can be a deterrent for its use in visible areas (**Figs. 1–4**).

Systematic syntheses of clinical trials' findings constitute the highest level of evidence and are essential to inform evidence-based guidelines and set the standard of care in all settings of dental practice. This article presents and discusses the findings of systematic reviews and metaanalysis of SDF as a treatment for caries arrest and prevention.

BACKGROUND

Silver compounds, especially silver nitrate, have been used in medicine to control infections for more than a century.[19] In dentistry, reports of use of silver nitrate are well-documented for caries inhibition[20] and, before the twentieth century, silver nitrate was firmly entrenched in the profession as a remedy for "hypersensitivity of dentin, erosion and pyorrhea, and as a sterilizing agent and caries inhibitor in deciduous as well as in permanent teeth."[21] Howe's solution (ammoniacal silver nitrate, 1917), was reported to disinfect caries lesions[22] and continued to be used for nearly one-half of a century as a sterilizing and disclosing agent for bacterial invasion of dentin[23,24] to avoid direct pulp exposures, to detect incipient lesions, and to disclose leftover carious dentin.[25]

The relationship of fluorides and caries prevention had been well-established through epidemiologic observations, chemical studies, animal experiments, and clinical trials beginning in the early decades of the twentieth century. It is now well-known that, when fluoride combines with enamel or dentin, it greatly reduces their solubility in acid, promotes remineralization, and results in a reduction of caries.[26]

The use of ammoniacal silver fluoride for the arrest of dental caries was pioneered by Drs Nishino and Yamaga in Japan,[27] who developed it to combine the actions of F⁻ and Ag⁺ and led to the approval of the first SDF product, Saforide (Bee Brand Medico Dental Co, Ltd, Osaka, Japan) in 1970.[28] Each milliliter of product contains 380 mg (38 w/v%) of $Ag(NH_3)_2F$. They described its effects for prevention and arrest of dental caries in children, prevention of secondary caries after restorations, and desensitization of hypersensitive dentin. They reported that it penetrated 20 μm into sound

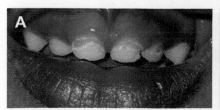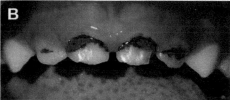

Fig. 1. (*A*) Enamel and dentin caries lesions in primary anterior teeth. (*B*) Same lesions showing staining after SDF treatment.

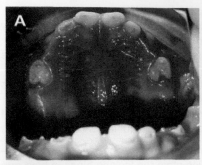
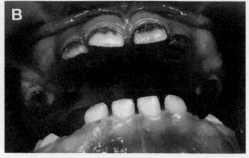

Fig. 2. (A) Caries lesions on enamel and dentin on young primary teeth. (B) Same lesions showing staining after SDF treatment.

enamel. In dentin, reported penetration of F⁻ was up to 50 to 100 μm and Ag⁺ went deeper than that, getting close to the pulp chamber.[28] They warned that because the agent stains the decalcified soft dentin black, its application should be confined to posterior teeth and gave specific instructions for its application.

Other similar products then became commercially available in other regions, like Silver Fluoride 40% in Australia (SCreighton Pharmaceuticals, Sydney),[29] Argentina (SDF 38% several brands), and Brazil (several SDF concentrations and brands).[30]

Since 2002,[31] the search for innovative approaches to address the caries pandemic resulted in the publication of many clinical trials of SDF efficacy (through comparison with no treatment), and its comparative effectiveness with other chemopreventive agents (eg, fluoride varnish [FV]), as well as other treatment interventions (eg, atraumatic restorative treatment [ART]). The results of these studies established the effectiveness of SDF as a caries arresting agent. In 2014, the US Food and Drug Administration approved SDF as a device for dentin desensitization in adults and, in 2015, the first commercial product became available in the United States: Advantage Arrest. Advantage Arrest (Elevate Oral Care, LLC, West Palm Beach, FL) is a 38% SDF solution (**Box 1**).

Manufacturer's instructions are limited to its approved use as a dentin desensitizer in adults. However, results from clinical trials conducted in many different countries on more than 3900 children have led investigators to develop recommendations for its use as a caries arrest medicament in children.[7,35]

In 2017, the American Academy of Pediatric Dentistry published a Guideline for the "Use of Silver Diamine Fluoride for Dental Caries Management in Children and Adolescents, Including Those with Special Health Care Needs."[36] This document encouraged the off-label adoption of this therapy for caries arrest, much as FV is used for

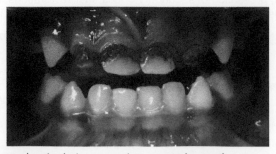

Fig. 3. Stained arrested caries lesions on primary anterior teeth.

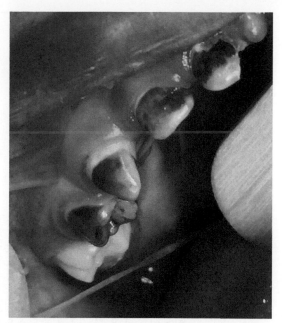

Fig. 4. Staining on non-cavitated and partially-cavitated enamel lesions.

caries prevention. In November 2016,[37] the US Food and Drug Administration granted SDF a breakthrough therapy status, which facilitates clinical trials of SDF for caries arrest to be carried out in the United States. Studies are currently underway that may result in the change of its labeling in the near future.[38]

Since 2009,[39] systematic reviews report on SDF's ability to arrest or prevent caries lesions. For this article, we reviewed systematic reviews reported in English and published or accepted for publication through March 2018. We identified 6 systematic reviews that met most of the PRISMA guidelines.[40] Their details can be found in **Table 1**. The outcomes reported in these reviews include efficacy (ability to arrest or prevent

---

Box 1
Manufacturer production description of silver-diamine fluoride 38%

Silver-Diamine Fluoride 38%	Professional tooth desensitizer
Desensitizing ingredient[32]	Aqueous silver diamine fluoride, 38.3%–43.2% w/v
Presentation[32,33]	Light-sensitive liquid with ammonia odor and blue coloring
	8 mL dropper-vials contain: approximately 250 drops; enough to treat 125 sites; a site is defined as up to 5 teeth; the unit-dose ampule contains 0.1 mL per ampule
Specific gravity[34]	1.25
Composition[34]	24%–27% silver
	7.5%–11.0% ammonia
	5%–6% fluoride (approximately 44,800 ppm)
	<1% blue coloring
	≤62.5% deionized water

Data from Refs.[32–34]

Table 1
Systematic reviews/metaanalysis on silver diamine fluoride trials

Author, Year	Outcome Measures	Studies Included and Max Follow-up Time Analyzed[a]		Dentitions Included/ Frequency of SDF Application[b]	Results
Rosenblatt et al,[39] 2009	Caries arrest and caries prevention	Systematic review only			SDF prevented fraction: caries arrest = 96.1%; caries prevention = 70.3%
		Chu,[31] 2002	30 mo	Primary max ant/q 12 mo	
		Llodra,[46] 2005	36 mo	Primary post teeth and First permanent molars/q 6 mo	
Horst et al,[35] 2016	Caries arrest and/or prevention	Systematic review only			Descriptive for each of the studies
		Chu,[31] 2002	30 mo	Primary max ant/q 12 mo	
		Llodra,[46] 2005	36 mo	Primary post teeth and First permanent molars/q 6 mo	
		Zhi,[45] 2012	24 mo	Primary ant and post/q 6 and q 12 mo	
		Yee,[64] 2009	24 mo	Primary ant and post/1 app only	
		Liu,[48] 2012	24 mo	Permanent first molars/q 12 mo	
		Monse,[50] 2012	18 mo	Permanent first molars/1 app only	
		Dos Santos,[65] 2014	12 mo	Primary ant and post/1 app only	
		Zhang,[66] 2013	24 mo	Root caries on elders/q 12 and q 24 mo	
		Tan,[67] 2010	36 mo	Root caries on elders/q 12 mo	

First author	Outcome	Studies included / description	Time	Teeth / application	Results
Gao et al,[18] 2016	Caries arrest in children	Metaanalysis included only SDF 38% at different time periods			Caries arrest rate of SDF 38% was 86% at 6 mo 81% at 12 mo 78% at 18 mo 71% at 30 mo or > Overall arrest was 81% (95% CI, 68%–89%; P<.001)
		Chu,[31] 2002	30 mo	Primary max ant/q 12 mo	
		Llodra,[46] 2005	36 mo	Primary post teeth and First permanent molars/q 6 mo	
		Zhi,[45] 2012	24 mo	Primary ant and post/q 6 and q 12 mo	
		Yee,[64] 2009	24 mo	Primary ant and post/1 app only	
		Wang, 1964 Chinese	18 mo	Primary ant and post/q 3 and q 4 mo	
		Yang, 2002 Chinese	6 mo	Primary teeth/1 app only	
		Ye, 1994 Chinese	12 mo	Primary teeth/1 app only	
		Fukumoto, 1997 Japanese	48 mo	Primary teeth/1app only	
Chibinski et al,[51] 2017	Control of caries progression in children after 12 mo follow-up	Metaanalysis included only studies with "low risk" of bias Evaluated at 12 mo results only (regardless of follow-up time) SDF vs control materials			Caries arrest was 89% higher than using active materials/placebo at 12 mo
		Duangthip,[43] 2016	12 mo	Primary ant and post/1 app/year or 3 app weekly at baseline	
		Zhi,[45] 2012	24 mo	Primary ant and post/q 6 and q 12 mo	
		NSP or SDF vs placebo			
		Dos Santos,[65] 2014 NSP	12 mo	Primary ant and post/1 app only	
		Seberol and Okte,[68] 2013 SDF (unpublished)	12 mo	Primary max ants only/1 app only	

(continued on next page)

Table 1
(continued)

Author, Year	Outcome Measures	Studies Included and Max Follow-up Time Analyzed[a]		Dentitions Included/ Frequency of SDF Application[b]	Results
Oliveira et al,[49] 2018	Prevention of new caries lesions in primary teeth	Metaanalysis included comparable studies evaluated at ≥24 mo			SDF applications reduce development of dentin lesions in treated and untreated primary teeth
		SDF vs placebo			PF: 77.5%; 95% CI, 67.8%–87.2%
		Chu,[31] 2002	30 mo	Primary max ant/q 12 mo	
		Llodra,[46] 2005	36 mo	Primary post teeth and First permanent molars/q 6 mo	
		SDF vs GIC			
		Dos Santos,[55] 2012	12 mo	Primary ant and post/1 app only	
Hendre et al,[53] 2017	Caries arrest and prevention in older adults	Systematic review only			Prevention:
		Tan,[67] 2010	36 mo	Root caries on elders/q 12 mo	PF of SDF vs placebo = 71% in 36-mo study
		n = 203			21% in a 24-mo study
		Zhang,[66] 2013	24 mo	Root caries on elders/q 12 and q 24 mo	Arrest:
		n = 227			PF of SDF vs placebo = 725% greater in 24-mo study
		Li,[58] 2016	30 mo	Root caries on elders/q 12 and q 24 mo	100% greater in 30 mo study
		n = 67			

Abbreviations: ant, anterior; app, reapplication; CI, confidence interval; NSP, nano-silver particles; PF, preventive fraction; post, posterior; SDF, silver-diamine fluoride.

[a] Number of subjects in published studies for SDF in children are included in **Table 2** n = listed in this table corresponds with the number of subjects in the study quoted not included in **Table 2**.

[b] q × mos refers to frequency of reapplication in months.

caries lesions) and comparative effectiveness (eg, equivalence or superiority when compared with other modalities such as ART and FV). Included reviews report on the primary and permanent dentitions of children and the permanent teeth on elderly populations. We consider each endpoint separately herein.

CURRENT EVIDENCE ON THE EFFICACY OF SILVER DIAMINE FLUORIDE FOR CARIES ARREST AND PREVENTION

In this section, we evaluate the results for SDF's efficacy for caries arrest as reported by the systematic reviews and metaanalysis included in **Table 1**. These systematic reviews used different perspectives to evaluate 17 prospective, parallel design, randomized, controlled clinical trials with a clearly defined outcome. As a result, and apparent from **Table 1**, many of the systematic reviews included refer to the same body of clinical trials, just updating results as additional studies became available. Details of each of the included clinical trials conducted on children and published in English are included in **Table 2**.

Taken together, the underlying clinical trials and systematic reviews indicate that SDF arrests caries in primary teeth and root caries in elders. and may prevent formation of new caries. Details on each of the outcomes measured on different dentitions and age groups are described in the following sections.

Caries Arrest on Primary Teeth in Children

All studies reach a similar conclusion supporting SDF's efficacy in arresting decay in primary teeth compared with no treatment and several other treatment modalities. Based on the Gao 2016 metaanalysis,[18] the proportion of caries arrest on primary teeth treated with different application protocols (1 application, annual, and biannual), and followed from 6 to 30 months, was 81% (95% confidence interval, 68%–89% $p<.001$). Chibinski and colleagues (2017)[51] reported that the caries arrest at 12 months promoted by SDF was 66% higher (41%–91%) than by other active material, but it was 154% higher (67%–85%) than by no treatment. Chibinski and associated[51] also reported a risk ratio of 1.66 (95% confidence interval, 1.41–1.96) when comparing SDF with active treatments, and a risk ratio of 2.54 (95% confidence interval, 1.67–3.85) when comparing SDF with no treatment.

It is apparent that the range of caries arrest is very wide, indicating that a proportion (that varies depending on the study) of the lesions receiving treatment will not become arrested. Several trials have stressed that in their results, anterior teeth have much higher rates of arrest than posterior teeth[41–45] As an example, one of the trials not included in the reviews, because it just published its 30-month results,[42] reports caries arrest by type of primary tooth using SDF 38% semiannually (**Box 2**).

In addition, this study, as have others,[44,45] found that lesions with visible plaque and large lesions had a lesser likelihood of arrest. The difference in arrest rates in children receiving applications twice per year versus once per year was small between 24 and 30 months in all teeth, but among children who received annual application, those with visible plaque had a lesser likelihood of having their lesions arrested. Fung and colleagues[42] conclude that, for children with poor oral hygiene, caries arrest rate can be increased by increasing the frequency of application from annually to semiannually.

Caries Arrest on Permanent Teeth in Children

The Rosenblatt review is the only one that addresses caries arrest in permanent teeth, and it is based on only 1 trial (Llodra and colleagues [2006][46]). They calculate a

Table 2
Description and clinical details of randomized control trials on children

	Chu et al,[31] 2002	Yee et al,[64] 2009	Zhi et al,[45] 2012	Dos Santos et al,[55] 2012	Duangthip et al,[44] 2018	Fung et al,[42] 2018	Llodra et al,[46] 2005	Braga et al,[47] 2009 2012	Liu et al,[48] 2009 2012	Monse et al,[50] 2012
Location	China	Nepal	China	Brazil	Hong Kong	China	Cuba	Brazil	China	Philippines
Dentition studied	Primary anterior only	Primary	Primary anterior and posterior	Primary	Primary anterior and posterior	Primary anterior and posterior	Primary cuspids, molars and permanent first molars	Permanent first molars	Permanent first molars	Permanent first molars
Caries effect studied	Arrest	Arrest	Arrest	Arrest	Arrest	Arrest	Arrest and prevention	Arrest	Prevention	Prevention
Groups compared	1. SDF (38%) 1×/y with caries removal 2. SDF (38%) 1×/y without caries removal 3. FV 5% 4× y with caries removal 4. FV 5% 4× y without caries removal 5. Water control	1. SDF (38%) 1× followed by tannic acid as reducing agent 2. SDF (38%) 1× alone 3. SDF (12%) 1× alone 4. No treatment	1. SDF (38%) 1×/y 2. SDF (38%) 2×/y 3. GI (Fuji VII) w/conditioner 1×/y	1. SDF(30%) 1× 2. ITR (Fuji IX) w/conditioner 1×.	1. SDF (30%) 1×/y 2. SDF (30%) 1×/week for 3 wk at baseline 3. FV (5%) 1×/wk for 3 wk at baseline	1. SDF (38%) 1×/y 2. SDF (38%) 2×/y 3. SDF (12%) 1×/y 4. SDF (12%) 2×/y	1. SDF (38%) 2×/y 2. No treatment	1. SDF (10%) 3× at 1-wk interval 2. GI (Fuji III) sealant 1× 3. Cross toothbrushing Noncavitated caries lesions On each child 1 molar was assigned to each group	1. SDF (38%) 1×/y 2. Resin sealant 3. 5% NaF varnish 2× y 4. Yearly placebo Deep fissures or non-cavitated early lesions Each child got same treatment in all molars	1. SDF (38%) 1× on sound and cavitated molars 2. ART (high-viscosity Ketac molar) on sound and cavitated molars 3. NT Some schools had tooth-brushing programs and some did not

Main findings	1. SDF was more effective than FV or control (65% arrested lesions for SDF groups vs 41% for FV groups vs 34% for control) 2. Caries removal had no effect 3. Control group developed more new caries than treatment groups	1. SDF was more effective than controls (31% arrested lesions for SDF vs 22% for SDF groups vs 12% vs 15% for control) 2. Tannic acid removal had no effect 3. Arrest benefit decreases over time	1. SDF and GI are equally effective (91% arrested lesions for SDF 2×/y vs 79% SDF 1×/y vs 82% GI 1×/y) 2. Increasing frequency of SDF (2×/y) increases caries arrest 3. Anterior teeth and buccal/lingual surfaces are more likely to become arrested	1. SDF was more effective than ITR (67% arrested lesions in SDF group vs 39% in control)	1. SDF 1×/y was more effective than SDF or FV 3 weekly applications at baseline (arrest of cavitated lesions: 48% SDF 1×/y vs 33% in group 2% and 34% with FV; for arrest of moderate lesions the 3 protocols were equally effective: 45% SDF 1×/y vs 44% in group 2% and 51% with FV)c	1. SDF 38% 2×/y was more effective than SDF 38% 1×/y, SDF 12% 2×/y or 1×/y (77% arrested lesions vs 67%, 59% and 55%, respectively)	1. SDF 2×/y was more effective for caries arrest than controls (85% arrested lesions with SDF vs 62% in control) 2. SDF was effective for caries reduction in both primary and permanent teeth (0.29 surfaces with new caries in SDF group vs 1.43 in control in primary teeth and 0.37 vs 1.06 in permanent molars)	1. SDF was more effective than toothbrushing or GI at 3 and 6 mo 2. All equally effective in controlling initial (non-cavitated) occlusal caries at 30 mo	1. The 3 active treatments are effective in caries prevention (progression of caries into dentin was 2.2% for SDF, 1.6% for sealant, 2.4% for FV vs 4.6% for control) 2. Control group developed more dentin caries than treatment groups	1. ART sealants were more effective than a single application of SDF (caries increment in the brushing group was: 0.08 for NT; 0.09 for SDF; 0.01 for sealants. In non-brushing group: 0.17 for NT; 0.12 for SDF; 0.06 for sealants) 2. Caries increment was lower in toothbrushing group

(continued on next page)

Table 2
(continued)

	Chu et al,[31] 2002	Yee et al,[64] 2009	Zhi et al,[45] 2012	Dos Santos et al,[55] 2012	Duangthip et al,[44] 2018	Fung et al,[42] 2018	Llodra et al,[46] 2005	Braga et al,[47] 2009	Liu et al,[48] 2012	Monse et al,[50] 2012
Additional findings	1. Arrested lesions looked black without changing parental satisfaction (93% of parents did not mention a difference)	1. Single SDF application prevented one-half of arrested surfaces at 6 mo from reverting to active lesions again over 24 mo 2. No complaints from parents or children to SDF	1. GI provides a more esthetic outcome. 2. Only 3.5% retention of GI after 24 mo still provides caries arrest 3. 45% of parents in all groups were satisfied with appearance	1. 43% of GIC fillings were lost at 6 mo and dentin was soft. 2. Higher rate of failure when GIC involved multiple surfaces.	1. Lesions in anterior teeth, buccal/lingual surfaces and lesions with no plaque had a higher chance to become arrested	1. Lesion site was significant, with lower anteriors having the highest rates of arrest followed by upper anteriors, lower posterior, and upper posterior 2. Lesions with visible plaque and large lesions had lower chance of becoming arrested	1. SDF showed more efficacy to arrest decay in deciduous teeth than permanent teeth	1. Retention rates for GI sealants were 32% at 6 mo and 9% at 30 mo 2. GI sealants were more time consuming that SDF application	1. Teeth with early caries at baseline were more likely to develop dentin caries after 24 mo 2. 46% sealant retention	1. Retention rate for sealants was 58% after 18 mo

SDF Clinical Application Protocol	Adverse effects	Duration of study (mo)	Baseline caries	Background F exposure
a Two treated groups had caries removal and 2 did not; a Does not specify SDF amount used or time of exposure	None	30	3.92 dmfs (active anterior lesions)	Low F exposure reported use of F toothpaste
a No caries removal; a One drop of SDF applied for 2 min to carious surfaces and dried with cotton pellet; a No food or drink for 1 h after	None	24	6.8 dmfs (active lesions)	Low F exposure Provided F toothpaste
a Minor excavation; a Does not specify SDF amount used or time of exposure; a No food or drink for 30 min after	None	24	5.1 dmft (3 random teeth/child)	Low F exposure low access to F toothpaste
a No caries removal; a Does not specify SDF amount used; a Cotton roll isolation, petroleum jelly on gingiva, SDF applied for 3 min and rinse and spit; a No food or drink for 1 h	None	12	3.8 dmft	Low F exposure access to F toothpaste
a No caries removal; a Does not specify SDF amount used or kind of isolation; a SDF rubbed for 10 s; • No food or drink for 30 min	None	30	4.4 dmft 6.7 dmfs	F water F toothpaste
a Does not specify SDF amount used, time of exposure, or kind of isolation	None	30	3.84 dmft 5.15 dmfs	Low F exposure F toothpaste
a Minor decay excavation on permanent molars only; a Does not specify SDF amount used, Cotton roll isolation, SDF applied for 3 min and wash for 30 s	0.1% Gingival irritation	36	3.2 dmft	Low F exposure + 0.2% NaF rinse in school every other week
a No caries removal; a Does not specify SDF amount used; a Cotton roll isolation and petroleum jelly on gingiva, SDF applied for 3 min, and wash for 30 s; a No food or drink for 1 h	None	30	Non-cavitated molar occlusal	Low F exposure Provided F toothpaste
a Does not specify SDF amount used, time of exposure, or whether it was rinsed or not; a Cotton roll isolation; a No food or drink for 30 min	None	24	No cavitated lesions	Low F exposure Provided F toothpaste
a Does not specify SDF amount used, SDF rubbed for 1 min followed by tannic acid, dried with cotton pellet, and covered with petroleum jelly; a Cotton roll isolation	None	18	At least 1 sound permanent molar	Low F exposure Provided F toothpaste

(continued on next page)

Table 2
(continued)

	Chu et al,[31] 2002	Yee et al,[64] 2009	Zhi et al,[45] 2012	Dos Santos et al,[55] 2012	Duangthip et al,[44] 2018	Fung et al,[42] 2018	Llodra et al,[46] 2005	Braga et al,[47] 2009	Liu et al,[48] 2012	Monse et al,[50] 2012
No. of subjects at baseline	375	976	212	91	371[b]	888	425	22 children, 66 molars	501	1016
No. of subjects at endpoint	308	634	181	?	309[b]	799	373	?	485	704
Examinations after baseline	×6 mo	1, 12, and 24 mo	×6 mo	×6 mo	×6 mo	×6 mo	×6 mo	3, 6, 12, 18 and 30 mo plus radiographs at 6, 12 and 30 mo	×6 mo	18 mo

Abbreviations: ART, atraumatic restorative treatment; dmfs, decayed/missing/filled surface; dmft, decayed/missing/filled teeth; FV, fluoride varnish; GI, glass ionomer; GIC, glass ionomer cements; NT, no treatment; SDF, silver diamine fluoride.

[a] Low F exposure = low F in the water, no other professionally applied fluorides or fluoride supplements.

[b] Number of subjects at baseline and endpoint reported on 30-mo results is different that numbers reported on 18-mo results.

[c] Cavitated lesions were International Caries Detection and Assessment System (ICDAS) 5 or 6; moderate lesions had no visible dentine and were ICDAS 3 or 4.

Modified from Crystal YO, Niederman R. Silver diamine fluoride treatment considerations in children's caries management. Pediatr Dent 2016;38(7):467–8; with permission.

Box 2	
Caries arrest by type of primary tooth using SDF 38% semiannually	
Overall arrest at 30 mo all teeth	75.0%
Lower anterior teeth	91.7%
Upper anterior teeth	85.6%
Lower posterior teeth	62.4%
Upper posterior teeth	57.0%

Data from Fung MHT, Duangthip D, Wong MCM, et al. Randomized clinical trial of 12% and 38% silver diamine fluoride treatment. J Dent Res 2018;97(2):171–8.

preventive fraction of 100% and number needed to treat of 1, basing their calculations on the mean number of arrested lesions was 0.1 in the SDF group and 0.2 in the control group. Llodra and associates (2006)[46] report that around 77% of treated caries that was active at baseline became inactive during the study, both in primary and in first permanent molars. Another small trial (on 22 children) studied caries arrest in permanent molars[47] (see **Table 2**) and found that SDF was more effective than toothbrushing or glass ionomer at 3 and 6 months, but they were all equally effective in controlling noncavitated lesions at 30 months No other systematic reviews were able to reach conclusions on caries arrest on permanent teeth in children owing to lack of solid evidence.

Caries Prevention in Children

The review undertaken by Rosenblatt and associates[39] evaluated SDF's potential for prevention using data from 2 trials. The trial from Llodra and colleagues (2006)[46] included primary and permanent molars and found that new caries lesion development (as a marker of caries prevention) in permanent teeth was significantly lower in the SDF group (0.4 new lesions) that in the water control group (1.1 new lesions) over 36 months. In primary teeth, the SDF groups averaged 0.3 new lesions versus 1.4 in the water control group. A trial conducted by Chu and associates (2002)[31] using only maxillary anterior teeth in preschool children found the mean number of new lesions over a period of 30 months in the SDF group was 0.47 versus 0.7 new lesions per year with 4 yearly applications of FV, versus 1.58 new lesions in the water control group. The review concludes that the preventive fraction for SDF was 70.3% (>60% on permanent teeth and >70% on primary teeth). Only 2 other clinical trials have studied caries preventive effect of SDF on permanent teeth. Liu and coworkers (2012)[48] found that proportions of pit/fissure sites with increased dentin caries treated with sealant, VF, and SDF were not significantly different at 24 months and they were all more effective than water control. Monse and associates (2012)[50] found that atraumatic treatment restorations sealants were more effective than a single application of SDF after 18 months. These 4 studies of permanent teeth have not been combined in a metaanalysis because they reported outcomes using different measures (number of teeth with new caries lesions or active lesions, in all surfaces vs only pit and fissure, and provide the data in different units of measurement [means and standard deviation vs number of events]).[51] No solid conclusions can be reached with such a small number of studies on permanent teeth in children.

In their recent systematic review and metaanalysis, Oliveira and colleagues[49] evaluated caries prevention for primary teeth and concluded that, when compared with placebo at 24 months or more, SDF decreased the development of dentin caries lesions in treated and untreated primary teeth with a preventive fraction of 77.5%.

Comparisons between SDF and FV concluded that SDF performed significantly better than FV at 18 and 30 months, and comparison between SDF and glass ionomer cements (GIC) showed that GIC was better than SDF at 12 months (not statistically significant). Both of these comparisons are weak because they are based on only 1 trial each.[31,55]

Because the trial from Llodra and associates[46] included only primary posterior teeth and newly erupted first molars, noncavitated lesions in pit and fissures may have been difficult to code and, therefore, may have been missed. In contrast, the trial from Chu and colleagues (2002)[31] studied only maxillary anterior teeth, where detection of new lesions would have been easier. Another problem making statements about the preventive effect of SDF on the whole dentition is that the trials included have reported new caries in only the teeth studied and not the whole dentition. Llodra and associates did not include any data on anterior teeth and the study by Chu and coworkers did not include any data on posterior teeth, even though they report that children had lesions and treatment in teeth not included in their study. Direct comparisons with the preventive effect of other modalities of fluoride applications are problematic, because those trials (on toothpaste of FV as an example) always report new caries in the whole dentition.

Caries Arrest and Prevention in the Elderly

In the only systematic review of SDF on adults, Hendre and colleagues[53] (2017) found no studies on coronal caries, but included 3 studies on root caries arrest and prevention. They found a preventive fraction for SDF of 24% in a 24-month study and 71% over a 36-month study. The preventive fraction for caries progression was 725% greater in a 24-month study and 100% greater than placebo in a 30-month study. From these findings, the investigators recommend the use of SDF for seniors who present increased root caries risk, used alone or in conjunction with oral hygiene education and other treatments. They go on to recommend SDF use to manage dentin sensitivity, based on a 7-day trial conducted on adults that was not included in their review.[52]

Only 1 other systematic review and metaanalysis included SDF in their study of noninvasive treatment of root caries lesions,[56] concluding that weak evidence indicates that SDF varnishes seem to be efficacious to decrease initiation of root caries. They based this conclusion on 2 studies (Tan 2010[67] and Zhang 2013[66]). However, because there seem to be some discrepancies in their methodology for the metaanalysis, we did not include their data in **Table 1**.

Side Effects and Toxicity

None of the reviews or trials report any acute side effects of the SDF used in the conditions of the individual trials on either children or adults. Minor side effects have been described as transient gingival irritation and metallic taste in a small number of participants. Only 1 published study on adults had an as aim to study gingival erythema 24 hours and 7 days after SDF application and found that, even when there was a very small number of participants who presented mild gingival erythema at 24 hours, there was no difference from baseline at 7 days.[52] This finding suggests that minor gingival irritations heal within a couple of days. A recent report from a clinical trial on young children[17] states that the prevalence of tooth and gum pain reported by parents was 6.6% 1 week after application, whereas gum swelling and gum bleaching were reported by 2.8% and 4.7%, respectively. SDF should not be used on lesions that are suspected of pulpal involvement because it will not prevent further progression of the infection into surrounding tissues[50] (**Fig. 5**).

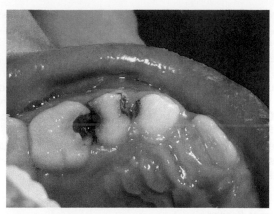

Fig. 5. Large lesion with cellulitis.

The main side effect of the use of SDF is the dark staining of the carious tooth tissue, which has raised concerns of parental satisfaction (see **Figs. 3** and **4**).[54] This study, which included 799 children in 37 kindergartens in Hong Kong,[17] reported that, although blackening of carious lesions was common with 38% SDF (66% to 76%), parental satisfaction with their children's dental appearance after 30 months was 71% to 62%. A US web-based survey that used photographs of carious teeth before and after SDF treatment found that parents considered staining on posterior teeth significantly more acceptable than on anterior teeth. However, even among those who found anterior staining unsightly, a significant number of parents would accept SDF treatment to avoid advanced behavioral techniques (like sedation or general anesthesia).[57] Most studies go on to recommend an appropriate informed consent so parents can understand the benefits and compromises of this therapy.[36]

SDF also temporarily stains skin and gingiva, requiring them to be handled so as to avoid contact with these tissues.

Many studies have suggested the use of potassium iodide applied after SDF application to control or reverse the staining. Some commercial products with both products are available (Riva Star, SDI, Baywater, Victoria, Australia). However, one of the trials for adults[58] reported that potassium iodide application had no effect in reducing the black stain on root caries, especially in the long term.

Although there has been no reported acute toxicity with SDF when used as recommended, the high concentration of fluoride has raised some concern,[59] especially with repeated applications on very young children. High concentrations of silver, a heavy metal, have raised similar concerns. Investigators who have conducted many of the clinical trials cited herein[60] have recommended that, although the amount of SDF applied is minute, precautions should be taken and multiple and frequent applications on young children should be avoided. The only study that reported on the pharmacokinetics of SDF after oral application[61] was done on only 6 adults over a period of 4 hours using 6 μL (about one-fifth of a drop) to treat 3 teeth on each subject. Their conclusion was that serum concentrations of fluoride and silver should pose little toxicity risk when used only occasionally in adults.

To date, there are no studies that have evaluated the long-term in vivo effects of silver on the oral microbiome or the total gastrointestinal microbiome. We do not know whether there are measurable traces of silver in saliva or plasma after SDF application and whether there could be long-term cumulative effects of silver in other organs.

Conclusions

SDF promises to be a therapy that could benefit many patients. In addition of the guideline for its use published by the American Academy of Pediatric Dentistry, the World Health Organization's 2016 report on Public Health Interventions against Early Childhood Caries, concluded that SDF can arrest dentine caries in primary teeth and prevent recurrence after treatment (very low evidence).[62] It recommends its use as an alternative procedure for tertiary prevention to reduce the negative impact of established disease (cavity) by restoring function and reducing disease-related complications and to improve the quality of life for children with early childhood caries.

Limitations of Current Research

Most of the systematic reviews and metaanalysis included for this article face the obstacles of having to compile data from clinical trials that have substantial differences in treatment protocols (1 application, yearly, or twice a year applications), concentration of SDF used, dentition studied, follow-up time, outcome measured (arrest or prevention), and the way they report their findings. Their reported figures differ depending on the number of studies included and how they group the studies to make their comparisons, which may affect the generalizability of their results.

It is also important to point out that all the clinical trials cited took place in school or community settings. Extrapolating recommendations from their results to clinical practice should take into consideration the availability of the patient for follow-up. Although SDF halts the caries process and desensitizes the decayed teeth, allowing for the implementation of better home care regimes, it does not restore form and function. As patient circumstances change, SDF-treated teeth may be restored as part of a comprehensive caries management plan.[36] SDF seems to be compatible with GIC and its effect on the bond strength of composite to treated dentin is still under study.[53] Laboratory observations report that SDF may also increase resistance of GIC and composite restorations to secondary caries.[63] Long-term clinical studies are required to recommend solid treatment protocols.

Future Research

The current reviews point to the need for studies that address the frequency and intensity of SDF used in conjunction with adjunctive preventive agents (eg, SDF with or without FV), the timing of application (eg, 1–4 times per year), and follow on restorative care (eg, glass ionomer or resin fillings). There may be differences in each of the foregoing strategies when comparing primary and permanent teeth, as well as anterior and posterior teeth. The longevity of arrest and prevention are unknown. Is SDF an agent that can be used, for example, 4 times per year, then terminated? Patient-centered outcomes also need to be addressed. The combination of clinical and patient centered outcomes will facilitate cost–benefit analysis and, thus, payment system improvement. Underlying all of this are generic biological questions, including the following: What is the impact on the oral microbiome? How does the interaction of the oral microbiome, the human genome, and SDF interact to affect caries? And finally, there is a clear need for the continued evolution of well-designed, randomized, clinical trials to produce studies with a low risk of bias during the planning, execution, and reporting of results. Standardization in the presentation of data between studies,[18,51] whether they focus on arrest or prevention, is imperative to be able to combine and translate the data into strong clinical guidelines. As indicated, clinicians need to know how to manage arrested lesions for longer periods, which is important for very young children and imperative for permanent teeth.

CLINICAL APPLICATIONS

From the current evidence available we can summarize that:

- 38% SDF solution is more effective than lower concentrations[18,42];
- No caries removal is necessary to achieve caries arrest[31];
- Twice a year application is more effective than yearly applications[18,42,45,51];
- Over longer periods (30 months), annual applications of SDF are more effective than 3 weekly applications at baseline[44];
- Application times ranging from 10 seconds[44] to 3 minutes[47,55] achieved various degrees of success that do not seem to be time dependent;
- Anterior teeth have higher rates of arrest than posterior teeth[41,42,44,45];
- Large lesions, occlusal lesions and those with visible plaque have less chances of arrest[41,42,44] (**Figs. 6** and **7**);
- Its use should be avoided in teeth with suspected pulpal involvement[50] (see **Fig. 5**); and
- Annual application of SDF seems to be effective for arrest and prevention of root caries on older adults who are capable of self-care. Multiple applications may benefit a more dependent and at-risk older population.[53]

With all age groups, clinicians should use their clinical judgment about application frequency based on individual caries risk factors, fluoride exposure, patient needs, and taking into consideration individual social determinants of health.

Clinical application is simple: the lips are protected with petroleum jelly (Vaseline) or lip balm, the tooth is isolated with cotton rolls, the lesion is cleaned of food debris and dried, and SDF is painted onto the clean lesion and allowed to air dry (**Fig. 8** and https://youtu.be/p9Tazwitcao). Rinsing after application does not seem to be necessary.

INDICATIONS

At the tooth level, SDF therapy for caries arrest is indicated for cavitated lesions on coronal or root surfaces that are not suspected to have pulpal involvement, are not

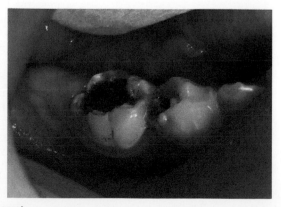

Fig. 6. Posterior arrest.

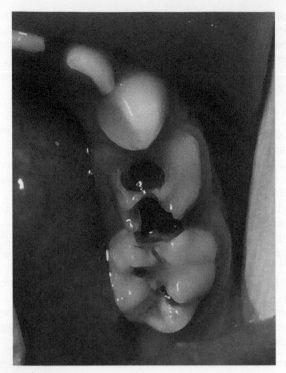

Fig. 7. Posterior partial arrest.

symptomatic, and are cleansable. Ideally, these conditions should be verified by radiographic evaluation.

PATIENT SELECTION AND MANAGEMENT

Patients who do not have immediate access to traditional restorative care can benefit from SDF therapy to arrest existing dentin caries lesions. This therapy is contraindicated on patients who report a silver allergy. Patients should be monitored closely to verify arrest of all lesions on a periodic basis based on risk factors; this is especially

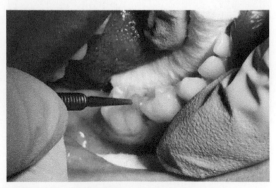

Fig. 8. Silver diamine fluoride application.

important when applied to permanent teeth. Follow-up should ideally include radiographic examination and the caries management plan should include plaque control, dietary counseling, combination of other fluoride modalities for caries prevention (like F varnish, fluoride gels, fluoride rinses and fluoride toothpaste) and sealants, depending on patient's age and individual situation. Follow-up on large lesions or lesions in hard-to-clean areas can be combined with the use of glass ionomer restorations or traditional restorative treatment, as patient circumstances allows.

REFERENCES

1. Sheiham A, Williams DM, Weyant RJ, et al. Billions with oral disease: a global health crisis–a call to action. J Am Dent Assoc 2015;146(12):861–4.
2. Petersen PE, Lennon MA. Effective use of fluorides for the prevention of dental caries in the 21st century: the WHO approach. Community Dent Oral Epidemiol 2004;32(5):319–21.
3. Petersen PE, Ogawa H. Prevention of dental caries through the use of fluoride–the WHO approach. Community Dent Health 2016;33(2):66–8.
4. Thompson FE, McNeel TS, Dowling EC, et al. Interrelationships of added sugars intake, socioeconomic status, and race/ethnicity in adults in the United States: National Health Interview Survey, 2005. J Am Diet Assoc 2009;109(8):1376–83.
5. Bagramian RA, Garcia-Godoy F, Volpe AR. The global increase in dental caries. A pending public health crisis. Am J Dent 2009;22(1):3–8.
6. Chaffee BW, Rodrigues PH, Kramer PF, et al. Oral health-related quality-of-life scores differ by socioeconomic status and caries experience. Community Dent Oral Epidemiol 2017;45(3):216–24.
7. Crystal YO, Niederman R. Silver diamine fluoride treatment considerations in children's caries management. Pediatr Dent 2016;38(7):466–71.
8. Horst JA. Silver fluoride as a treatment for dental caries. Adv Dent Res 2018; 29(1):135–40.
9. Gregory D, Hyde S. Root caries in older adults. J Calif Dent Assoc 2015;43(8): 439–45.
10. Featherstone JDB. Remineralization, the natural caries repair process–the need for new approaches. Adv Dent Res 2009;21:4–7.
11. Niederman R, Feres M, Ogunbodede E. Dentistry. In: Debas HT, Donkor P, Gawande A, et al, editors. Essential surgery: disease control priorities. Washington, DC: The 2015 International Bank for Reconstruction and Development/The World Bank.; 2015. p. 173–95.
12. Mei ML, Li QL, Chu CH, et al. Antibacterial effects of silver diamine fluoride on multi-species cariogenic biofilm on caries. Ann Clin Microbiol Antimicrob 2013; 12:4.
13. Mei ML, Ito L, Cao Y, et al. Inhibitory effect of silver diamine fluoride on dentine demineralisation and collagen degradation. J Dent 2013;41(9):809–17.
14. Chu CH, Lo EC. Microhardness of dentine in primary teeth after topical fluoride applications. J Dent 2008;36(6):387–91.
15. Mei ML, Nudelman F, Marzec B, et al. Formation of fluorohydroxyapatite with silver diamine fluoride. J Dent Res 2017;96(10):1122–8.
16. Mei ML, Chu CH, Low KH, et al. Caries arresting effect of silver diamine fluoride on dentine carious lesion with S. mutans and L. acidophilus dual-species cariogenic biofilm. Med Oral Patol Oral Cir Bucal 2013;18(6):e824–31.
17. Duangthip D, Fung MHT, Wong MCM, et al. Adverse effects of silver diamine fluoride treatment among preschool children. J Dent Res 2018;97(4):395–401.

18. Gao SS, Zhao IS, Hiraishi N, et al. Clinical trials of silver diamine fluoride in arresting caries among children: a systematic review. JDR Clin Transl Res 2016;1(3):201–10.
19. Higginbottom J. On the use of the nitrate of silver in the cure of erysipelas. Prov Med Surg J 1847;11(17):458–60.
20. Stebbins EA. What value has argenti nitras as a therapeutic agent in dentistry? Int Dent J 1891;12:661–70.
21. Seltzer S, Werther L. Conservative silver nitrate treatment of borderline cases of deep dental caries. J Am Dent Assoc 1941;28(October):1586–91.
22. Howe PR. A method of sterilizing and at the same time impregnating with a metal affected dentinal tissue. Dental Cosmos 1917;59(9):891–904.
23. Seltzer S. The comparative value of various medicaments in cavity sterilization. J Am Dent Assoc 1941;28(November):1844–52.
24. Seltzer S. Medication and pulp protection for the deep cavity in a child's tooth. J Am Dent Assoc 1949;39(August):148–57.
25. Zander HA. Use of silver nitrate in the treatment of caries. J Am Dent Assoc 1941; 28(8):1260–7.
26. Bibby BG. Use of fluorine in the prevention of dental caries. J Am Dent Assoc 1944;31(3):228–36.
27. Nishino M, Yoshida S, Sobue S, et al. Effect of topically applied ammoniacal silver fluoride on dental caries in children. J Osaka Univ Dent Sch 1969;9:149–55.
28. Yamaga R, Nishino M, Yoshida S, et al. Diamine silver fluoride and its clinical application. J Osaka Unic Dent Sch 1972;12(20):1–10.
29. Gotjamanos T. Pulp response in primary teeth with deep residual caries treated with silver fluoride and glass ionomer cement ('atraumatic' technique). Aust Dent J 1996;41(5):328–34.
30. Mei ML, Chin-Man Lo E, Chu CH. Clinical use of silver diamine fluoride in dental treatment. Compend Contin Educ Dent 2016;37(2):93–8 [quiz: 100].
31. Chu CH, Lo ECM, Lin HC. Effectiveness of silver diamine fluoride and sodium fluoride varnish in arresting dentin caries in Chinese pre-school children. J Dent Res 2002;81(11):767–70.
32. ElevateOralCare. Advantage arrest SDF 38% bottle. Available at: http://www.elevateoralcare.com/dentist/AdvantageArrest/Advantage-Arrest-Silver-Diamine-Fluoride-38. Accessed November 1, 2018.
33. ElevateOralCare. Advantage arrest: SDF 38% product package insert. Available at: http://www.elevateoralcare.com/site/images/AA_PI_040715.pdf. Accessed November 1, 2018.
34. ElevateOralCare. Safety data sheet. Advantage arrest SDF 38%. Available at: http://www.elevateoralcare.com/site/images/AASDS082415.pdf. Accessed November 1, 2018.
35. Horst JA, Ellenikiotis H, Milgrom PL. UCSF protocol for caries arrest using silver diamine fluoride: rationale, indications and consent. J Calif Dent Assoc 2016; 44(1):16–28.
36. Crystal YO, Marghalani AA, Ureles SD, et al. Use of silver diamine fluoride for dental caries management in children and adolescents, including those with special health care needs. Pediatr Dent 2017;39(5):135–45.
37. ElevateOralCare. The silver bulletin 1. 2017. Available at: http://www.elevateoralcare.com/Landing-Pages/silverbulletinv1. Accessed September 16, 2018.
38. Phase III RCT of the effectiveness of silver diamine fluoride in arresting cavitated caries lesions NIH report. Project Information; 2017.

39. Rosenblatt A, Stamford TC, Niederman R. Silver diamine fluoride: a caries "silver-fluoride bullet". J Dent Res 2009;88(2):116–25.
40. Moher D, Liberati A, Tetzlaff J, et al. Preferred reporting items for systematic reviews and meta-analyses: the PRISMA statement. J Clin Epidemiol 2009;62(10):1006–12.
41. Fung MHT, Duangthip D, Wong MCM, et al. Arresting dentine caries with different concentration and periodicity of silver diamine fluoride. JDR Clin Transl Res 2016;1(2):143–52.
42. Fung MHT, Duangthip D, Wong MCM, et al. Randomized clinical trial of 12% and 38% silver diamine fluoride treatment. J Dent Res 2018;97(2):171–8.
43. Duangthip D, Chu CH, Lo EC. A randomized clinical trial on arresting dentine caries in preschool children by topical fluorides–18 month results. J Dent 2016;44:57–63.
44. Duangthip D, Wong MCM, Chu CH, et al. Caries arrest by topical fluorides in preschool children: 30-month results. J Dent 2018;70:74–9.
45. Zhi QH, Lo EC, Lin HC. Randomized clinical trial on effectiveness of silver diamine fluoride and glass ionomer in arresting dentine caries in preschool children. J Dent 2012;40(11):962–7.
46. Llodra JC, Rodriguez A, Ferrer B, et al. Efficacy of silver diamine fluoride for caries reduction in primary teeth and first permanent molars of schoolchildren: 36-month clinical trial. J Dent Res 2005;84(8):721–4.
47. Braga MM, Mendes FM, De Benedetto MS, et al. Effect of silver diamine fluoride on incipient caries lesions in erupting permanent first molars: a pilot study. J Dent Child (Chic) 2009;76(1):28–33.
48. Liu BY, Lo EC, Chu CH, et al. Randomized trial on fluorides and sealants for fissure caries prevention. J Dent Res 2012;91(8):753–8.
49. Oliveira BRA, Veitz-Keenan A, Niederman R. The effect of silver diamine fluoride in preventing caries in the primary dentition: a systematic review and meta-analysis. Caries Res 2018;53(1):24–32.
50. Monse B, Heinrich-Weltzien R, Mulder J, et al. Caries preventive efficacy of silver diamine fluoride (SDF) and ART sealants in a school-based daily fluoride toothbrushing program in the Philippines. BMC Oral Health 2012;12:52.
51. Chibinski AC, Wambier LM, Feltrin J, et al. Silver diamine fluoride has efficacy in controlling caries progression in primary teeth: a systematic review and meta-analysis. Caries Res 2017;51(5):527–41.
52. Castillo JL, Rivera S, Aparicio T, et al. The short-term effects of diamine silver fluoride on tooth sensitivity: a randomized controlled trial. J Dent Res 2011;90(2):203–8.
53. Hendre AD, Taylor GW, Chavez EM, et al. A systematic review of silver diamine fluoride: effectiveness and application in older adults. Gerodontology 2017;34(4):411–9.
54. Nelson T, Scott JM, Crystal YO, et al. Silver diamine fluoride in pediatric dentistry training programs: survey of graduate program directors. Pediatr Dent 2016;38(3):212–7.
55. dos Santos VE Jr, de Vasconcelos FMN, Ribeiro AG, et al. Paradigm shift in the effective treatment of caries in schoolchildren at risk. Int Dent J 2012;62(1):47–51.
56. Wierichs RJ, Meyer-Lueckel H. Systematic review on noninvasive treatment of root caries lesions. J Dent Res 2015;94(2):261–71.
57. Crystal YO, Janal MN, Hamilton DS, et al. Parental perceptions and acceptance of Silver Diamine Fluoride (SDF) staining. J Am Dent Assoc 2017;148(7):510–8.e4.

58. Li R, Lo EC, Liu BY, et al. Randomized clinical trial on arresting dental root caries through silver diamine fluoride applications in community-dwelling elders. J Dent 2016;51:15–20.
59. Gotjamanos T. Safety issues related to the use of silver fluoride in paediatric dentistry. Aust Dent J 1997;42(3):166–8.
60. Chu CH, Lo EC. Promoting caries arrest in children with silver diamine fluoride: a review. Oral Health Prev Dent 2008;6(4):315–21.
61. Vasquez E, Zegarra G, Chirinos E, et al. Short term serum pharmacokinetics of diamine silver fluoride after oral application. BMC Oral Health 2012;12:60.
62. Phantumvanit P, Makino Y, Ogawa H, et al. WHO global consultation on public health intervention against early childhood caries. Community Dent Oral Epidemiol 2018;46(3):280–7.
63. Mei ML, Zhao IS, Ito L, et al. Prevention of secondary caries by silver diamine fluoride. Int Dent J 2016;66(2):71–7.
64. Yee R, Holmgren C, Mulder J, et al. Efficacy of silver diamine fluoride for Arresting Caries Treatment. J Dent Res 2009;88(7):644–7.
65. dos Santos VE Jr, Vasconcelos Filho A, Ribeiro Targino AG, et al. A New "Silver-Bullet" to treat caries in children - Nano Silver Fluoride: A randomised clinical trial. Journal of Dentistry 2014;42(8):945–51.
66. Zhang W, McGrath C, Lo EC, et al. Silver diamine fluoride and education to prevent and arrest root caries among community-dwelling elders. Caries Res 2013; 47(4):284–90.
67. Tan HP, Lo EC, Dyson JE, et al. A randomized trial on root caries prevention in elders. J Dent Res 2010;89(10):1086–90.
68. Seberol EO. Z. Caries arresting effect of silver diamine fluoride on primary teeth. J Dent Res. 2013;Vol. 92 (Spec Iss C) abstract 48 (World Congress on Preventive Dentistry).

Evidence-Based Update on Diagnosis and Management of Gingivitis and Periodontitis

Satish Kumar, DMD, MDSc, MS

KEYWORDS

- Chronic periodontitis • Aggressive periodontitis • Periodontal diagnosis
- Periodontal therapy

KEY POINTS

- Dysbiosis between microbes and the host immune system altered with environmental and genetic factors is the current understanding of etiopathogenesis of chronic periodontitis.
- Management of periodontitis should involve an individualized risk assessment and treatment plan that include appropriate risk factor mitigation, such as control of diabetes, smoking cessation, among others.
- Prevention of gingivitis and consequently periodontitis involves maintaining meticulous oral hygiene by tooth brushing twice daily with preferably powered toothbrushes and fluoridated tooth paste, flossing, use of interdental brushes, and essential oil mouth rinses.
- Professional management of periodontitis include scaling and root planing with beneficial effects noted using adjuncts in specific situations.
- Persistent periodontitis after nonsurgical therapy will necessitate surgical periodontal therapy. Resective or regenerative periodontal therapies will aid in the elimination of remaining periodontitis and, hence, in retention of teeth.

PERIODONTAL DISEASE: DEFINITION

Periodontal disease comprises all diseases that affect the periodontium: gingiva, periodontal ligament, cementum, and alveolar bone. These diseases range from gingivitis to viral infections to tumors. Hence, the cause ranges from a simple, unifactorial agent, such as herpes simplex virus, to complex, multifactorial bacteria-host immune system–mediated dysbiosis.[1]

UPDATE IN DIAGNOSIS CLASSIFICATION

In 2015, the American Academy of Periodontology (AAP), published a focused update to the AAP's 1999 classification of periodontal diseases[2] on 3 issues regarding the

Disclosure Statement: The author has nothing to disclose.
A.T. Still University, Arizona School of Dentistry and Oral Health, 5855 E Still Circle, Mesa, AZ 85296, USA
E-mail address: satishkumar@atsu.edu

diagnosis of periodontitis.[3] They include further clarifications on the differences between chronic and aggressive periodontitis, guidelines on determining the severity of periodontitis, and, localized versus generalized periodontitis. More recently, in June 2018, the AAP in collaboration with the European Federation of Periodontology published a series of review and consensus articles by experts around the world in periodontics and implant dentistry to update the periodontal disease classification.[4–8] Several major updates have been proposed through this series. One of the major changes in this update is the proposal of combining chronic and aggressive periodontitis as a single-entity periodontitis exhibiting different phenotypes.[9] For the sake of familiarity by dental practitioners and the relatively recent release of the updated classification, this review focuses on the review of gingivitis (dental-biofilm–induced gingivitis), chronic periodontitis (slow to moderate rates of disease progression), and aggressive periodontitis (rapid rate of disease progression). The readers are recommended to the cited references for further understanding of the updated 2017 classification.

Chronic and Aggressive Periodontitis

In general, chronic periodontitis affects adults and corresponds to the amount of local factors, mainly plaque/calculus. It tends to progress slowly with periods of exacerbation. Systemic diseases, such as diabetes, and environmental risk factors, such as smoking, impact the severity of chronic periodontitis (**Fig. 1**). In contrast, aggressive periodontitis affects younger individuals (<25 years of age) with familial aggregation and the striking feature being rapid destruction of attachment and bone with little or no microbial deposits. Most patients with aggressive periodontitis are otherwise healthy systemically (**Fig. 2**). According to the updated 2017 classification, both cases in **Figs. 1** and **2** would be called periodontitis but will have different stages and grades.[10]

PERIODONTAL DISEASE: PREVALENCE AND BURDEN OF TOOTH LOSS

The prevalence of periodontal disease in the United States was estimated using the National Health and Nutrition Examination Survey data.[11] Full-mouth periodontal examination was done in this population measuring periodontal pockets and gingival recession (distance between free gingival margin to cementoenamel junction) in 6 sites for all teeth except the third molars.[12,13] The prevalence of periodontitis in the United States was estimated to be 45.9% during the period of 2009 to 2012 with severe periodontitis attributed to 8.9% of the American people. Severe periodontitis affects about 11.2% globally.[14] It is unfortunate that significant gaps in knowledge exist among the public regarding periodontal disease.[15]

SYSTEMIC DISEASE CONNECTION

Numerous studies over the last few decades have studied associations between periodontitis and systemic diseases as risk factors.[16] Although there is an established association between certain diseases, such as diabetes,[17] obesity,[18] and cardiovascular diseases,[19] most associations are not very strong. It is important to realize that managing periodontal disease for its own right is important because of the poor quality of life associated with tooth loss.[20,21] Association with systemic diseases, although very important to study to reduce the overall morbidity associated with both periodontitis and systemic diseases, should not distract the focus on managing periodontal disease for its own sake as the second most common oral disease after dental caries. Insufficient or low-quality evidence makes it difficult to understand whether periodontal

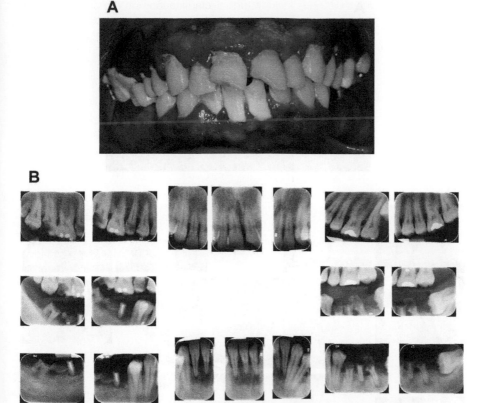

Fig. 1. (*A*) A 52-year-old man presenting with generalized microbial deposits and gingival inflammation. The local factors are consistent with clinical parameters of deeper probing depths, bleeding on probing, clinical attachment loss, mobility, and furcation. (*B*) Full-mouth series of radiographs show mild to severe bone loss along with multiple periapical radiolucencies due to pulpal disease. The diagnosis is consistent with generalized severe chronic periodontitis.

treatment has any positive effects on improving diabetes[22] or reducing low birth weight, preterm weight, or adverse obstetric outcomes.[23] Tooth loss is associated with significant reductions in quality of life.[24]

ETIOPATHOGENESIS

It has been long known that dental plaque and calculus initiate gingival inflammation (gingivitis)[25] and that given sustained presence of this gingival inflammation can eventually, in many cases, progress to destruction of underlying connective tissue and alveolar bone (periodontitis).[26,27] The interesting observation has been that not all gingivitis progressed in the same manner despite identical local factors. Individual variability in the host response to local factors plays a crucial role in this difference.[28] Today, it is known that the balance between host and bacteria determines the state of health, and the loss of this balance leads to what is termed dysbiosis and state of disease (referred to as polymicrobial synergy and dysbiosis model).[29] Certain keystone pathogens, such as *Porphyromonas gingivalis*, even in low

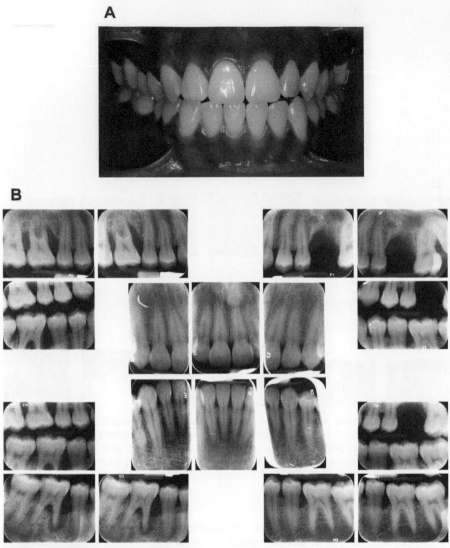

Fig. 2. (*A*) A 22-year-old man presenting with almost complete absence of microbial deposits. This presentation was inconsistent with clinical parameters of deeper probing depths, bleeding on probing, clinical attachment loss, and mobility mainly associated with first molars. (*B*) Full-mouth series of radiographs show severe bone loss along the remaining first molars. The diagnosis is consistent with localized aggressive periodontitis.

abundance, has been shown to lead to dysbiosis.[30] Herpes viruses have been implicated in the cause of periodontitis.[31] A recent meta-analysis using 12 case-control studies found herpes simplex virus type 1 and human cytomegalovirus to be significantly associated with aggressive periodontitis.[32] The investigators caution against the heterogeneity among the studies while interpreting these findings. Also, the association between Epstein-Barr virus (EBV) and herpes simplex virus type 2 was inconclusive because of insufficient evidence and publication bias. According to another meta-analysis, EBV was frequently detected in periodontal pockets of

5 mm or greater.[33] Besides the microbial-host interactions in disease onset and progression, genetics,[34] epigenetics,[35] diabetes,[36] and smoking (a major lifestyle risk factor)[37] have all been shown to have a major impact on disease onset and progression.

RISK ASSESSMENT

Using personalized risk assessment tools, such as the periodontal risk assessment[38] and the periodontal risk calculator (PRC),[39] may lead to better risk assessment and counseling of patients for better periodontal health.[40] The PRC takes the following information into consideration to calculate periodontal disease progression: *'patient age; smoking history; diabetes diagnosis; history of periodontal surgery; pocket depth; bleeding on probing; restorations below the gingival margin; root calculus; radiographic bone height; furcation involvements; and vertical bone lesions.'*[41] For example, a recent systematic review clearly showed that teeth with furcal involvement had a higher risk of tooth loss. However, the same study showed that periodontal therapy on furcal involved teeth reduced the loss of teeth.[42] Smoking counseling and dietary interventions to improve periodontal outcomes has been shown to be effective, and dental practitioners should include this as part of discussion from the initial visit and through periodontal maintenance.[43] Genetic risk assessment, such as interleukin-1 genetic tests, have been attempted in the past and have not been shown to be clinically useful yet.[41,44,45]

PREVENTION AND MANAGEMENT

Tooth brushing reduces dental plaque.[46] Powered toothbrushes,[47] especially the oscillating-rotating type,[48] have been shown to improve plaque levels and gingivitis. Similar findings were also observed with gingival index and gingival bleeding in patients undergoing orthodontic treatment. Nine randomized controlled trials were included in a meta-analysis for this finding.[49] For removal of plaque from interdental areas, using interdental brushes has been shown to be very effective.[50–52] Waterjets have also been shown to be effective recently in a meta-analysis along with interdental brushing.[53] Essential oil containing mouthwashes[54,55] and chlorhexidine mouth rinses[56] have been shown to be effective in reducing gingivitis and plaque levels. For patients with oral malodor, mouth rinses containing a combination of chlorhexidine, cetylpyridinium chloride, and zinc or a combination of cetylpyridinium chloride and zinc chloride have been found helpful.[57] Probiotics used as an adjunct to scaling and root planing (SRP) have been shown to have a short-term benefit in the management of chronic periodontitis.[58] Much of the evidence has been shown in the probiotic *Lactobacillus reuteri* (*L reuteri*).[59,60]

The 11th European Workshop on Periodontology published recommendations on the prevention of periodontal and peri-implant diseases in 2015 as a consensus report, which was also endorsed by the AAP. These recommendations were developed from 16 systematic reviews and meta-reviews of the same.[37,61–63]

For the management of gingivitis[64]

- Brushing twice daily for 2 minutes with powered toothbrushes using a fluoridated toothpaste
- Flossing in teeth with tighter contacts around healthy gingival tissue
- Using interproximal brushing especially around inflamed gingival tissue where flossing may cause trauma
- Using chemical plaque control agents like mouth rinses

American Dental Association's Clinical Practice Guideline

The American Dental Association (ADA) has recently published a systematic review and meta-analysis on the nonsurgical management of chronic periodontitis.[65] This review aided in the development of clinical practice guidelines[66] that outline recommendations based on the best available evidence on various nonsurgical modalities and expert opinion when evidence was unavailable or unclear. The clinical recommendations can be obtained from the ADA Web site.[67] The investigators looked at the net benefit for all nonsurgical treatment modalities balancing the benefits versus potential harms. The clinical relevance was estimated based on the clinical attachment level (CAL) improvement. The clinical effect was judged as zero, small, moderate, and substantial if the CAL were 0 to 0.2 mm, greater than 0.2 to 0.4, greater than 0.4 to 0.6, and greater than 0.6, respectively. It must be noted that the average CAL improvement noted for all recommended treatments ranged between 0.24 mm to 0.64 mm. The clinical recommendations were in favor of SRP without any adjuncts as well as SRP with systemic subantimicrobial-dose doxycycline. The specific dosage recommended for moderate to severe chronic periodontitis was doxycycline 20 mg twice a day for 3 to 9 months. Other adjuncts that were recommended with weak strength of evidence were SRP with systemic antimicrobials, locally delivered antimicrobials (chlorhexidine chips), and photodynamic therapy (PDT) using diode lasers. Expert opinion recommendations included SRP with locally delivered antimicrobials, namely, doxycycline hyclate gel and minocycline microspheres. It should be noted that this guideline concluded that there was no net benefit from using diode (non-PDT),[68] Nd:YAG,[69] and erbium lasers. Another systematic review has concluded that the evidence is insufficient for the use of lasers as an adjunct in periodontal resective or regenerative surgeries.[70]

Systemic Antibiotics

Systemic antibiotics have been shown to be helpful in the management of chronic periodontitis as an adjunct to SRP. The combination of amoxicillin and metronidazole used short-term along with SRP especially in patients with a periodontal pocket depth of 6 mm or more has been clinically significant.[71] The same combination has also been shown to be useful in the management of aggressive periodontitis.[72] Azithromycin has been also shown to improve the clinical outcomes when used as an adjunct to SRP.[73,74] In addition, azithromycin has been shown to be very effective in the management of cyclosporine-induced gingival overgrowth.[75] Full-mouth disinfection including the use of antibiotics/antiseptics or full-mouth scaling within 24 hours have been studied extensively as an alternate to quadrant-wise SRP. A recent systematic review has not found a significant difference in these modalities.[76] Host modulation therapy using antiinflammatory medications, such as nonsteroidal antiinflammatory drugs, have been shown to reduce gingivitis but are not recommended in clinical practice because of the limited quality of evidence and known side effects.[77]

Periodontal Surgical Therapy

When initial nonsurgical therapy using SRP and other adjuncts fail to resolve periodontitis during reevaluation, periodontal surgical therapy is indicated. Surgical therapy has been shown to be beneficial at an average probing depth of 5.4 mm.[78] Osseous surgery has been shown to improve CAL gain compared with SRP in deeper periodontal pockets of 7 mm or greater.[79] In certain scenarios, such as intrabony periodontal defects with well-contained osseous walls, regenerative periodontal therapy can be beneficial.[80]

Supportive Periodontal Therapy

Supportive periodontal therapy to maintain the improved periodontal health after active periodontal therapy has been shown to reduce the risk of tooth loss.[81,82] Oral hygiene instructions for patients is usually effective among motivated patients. Behavioral interventions, such as motivational interviewing, have been shown to be very effective in improving periodontal outcomes. Motivational interviewing involves personalizing the oral hygiene needs and communicating in a way that brings out the intrinsic motivation among patients.[83]

Personalized Care

Several factors discussed thus far, such as dysbiosis, genetic, environmental, and behavioral risk factors, among others, lead to interindividual and intraindividual variability in periodontal disease onset, progression pattern, and response to therapy. Prognostication of periodontally compromised teeth becomes challenging due to the multifactorial and complex nature of risk factors. Prognostication scoring systems, such as the Miller-McEntire scoring system for molars, may be useful for assessing prognosis.[84] Hence, personalized maintenance protocols based on risk factors should be established. Dental practitioners must become comfortable with general health risk assessments with interprofessional collaboration to improve not only periodontal health but also general health, such as by participating in smoking cessation and dietary modifications for weight control, among others.[85–87] Specific recall intervals, such as every 3 to 6 months, do not have strong support of evidence.[88]

SUMMARY

- Chronic periodontitis is a chronic inflammatory disease initiated by microbial biofilm and mediated by dysbiosis between the microbial biofilm and host inflammatory response.
- Aggressive periodontitis can be differentiated from chronic periodontitis by the rapid destruction of periodontium in a relatively short time in a relatively younger individuals (<25 years of age) with minimal presence or at times absence of calculus. Familial aggregation is common in aggressive periodontitis.
- Severe periodontitis affects about 11% of the world's population.
- Certain systemic diseases, such as diabetes, have a strong established bidirectional relationship with periodontitis.
- Management of periodontitis should be focused on for its consequences of tooth loss and related loss of quality of life rather than merely its association with a plethora of systemic diseases and their consequences.
- Dysbiosis between microbes and the host immune system altered with environmental and genetic factors is the current understanding of etiopathogenesis of chronic periodontitis. This process is complex and multifactorial. Hence, prediction of disease progression and response to treatment can vary tremendously within individuals and within the same individual.
- Management of periodontitis should involve an individualized risk assessment and treatment plan that include appropriate risk factor mitigation, such as control of diabetes and smoking cessation, among others.
- Prevention of gingivitis and consequently periodontitis involves maintaining meticulous oral hygiene by tooth brushing twice daily preferably with powered toothbrushes and fluoridated tooth paste, flossing, use of interdental brushes, and essential oil mouth rinses.

- Professional management of periodontitis includes SRP with beneficial effects noted using adjuncts in specific situations. Adjuncts include systemic antibiotics, systemic subantimicrobial-dose doxycycline, locally delivered antimicrobials (chlorhexidine chips, doxycycline hyclate gel, and minocycline microspheres), and PDT using diode lasers.

REFERENCES

1. Kinane DF, Stathopoulou PG, Papapanou PN. Periodontal diseases. Nat Rev Dis Primers 2017;3:17038.
2. 1999 International workshop for a classification of periodontal diseases and conditions. Papers. Oak Brook, Illinois, October 30-November 2, 1999. Ann Periodontol 1999;4(1):i, 1-112.
3. American Academy of Periodontology task force report on the update to the 1999 classification of periodontal diseases and conditions. J Periodontol 2015;86(7): 835–8.
4. G Caton J, Armitage G, Berglundh T, et al. A new classification scheme for periodontal and peri-implant diseases and conditions - introduction and key changes from the 1999 classification. J Periodontol 2018;89(Suppl 1):S1–8.
5. Chapple ILC, Mealey BL, Van Dyke TE, et al. Periodontal health and gingival diseases and conditions on an intact and a reduced periodontium: consensus report of workgroup 1 of the 2017 world workshop on the classification of periodontal and peri-implant diseases and conditions. J Periodontol 2018;89(Suppl 1): S74–84.
6. Papapanou PN, Sanz M, Buduneli N, et al. Periodontitis: consensus report of workgroup 2 of the 2017 World Workshop on the classification of periodontal and peri-implant diseases and conditions. J Periodontol 2018;89(Suppl 1): S173–82.
7. Jepsen S, Caton JG, Albandar JM, et al. Periodontal manifestations of systemic diseases and developmental and acquired conditions: consensus report of workgroup 3 of the 2017 World Workshop on the classification of periodontal and peri-implant diseases and conditions. J Periodontol 2018;89(Suppl 1):S237–48.
8. Berglundh T, Armitage G, Araujo MG, et al. Peri-implant diseases and conditions: consensus report of workgroup 4 of the 2017 World Workshop on the classification of periodontal and peri-implant diseases and conditions. J Periodontol 2018; 89(Suppl 1):S313–8.
9. Fine DH, Patil AG, Loos BG. Classification and diagnosis of aggressive periodontitis. J Periodontol 2018;89(Suppl 1):S103–19.
10. Tonetti MS, Greenwell H, Kornman KS. Staging and grading of periodontitis: framework and proposal of a new classification and case definition. J Periodontol 2018;89(Suppl 1):S159–72.
11. Eke PI, Dye BA, Wei L, et al. Update on prevalence of periodontitis in adults in the United States: NHANES 2009 to 2012. J Periodontol 2015;86(5):611–22.
12. Page RC, Eke PI. Case definitions for use in population-based surveillance of periodontitis. J Periodontol 2007;78(Suppl 7S):1387–99.
13. Eke PI, Dye BA, Wei L, et al. Prevalence of periodontitis in adults in the United States: 2009 and 2010. J Dent Res 2012;91(10):914–20.
14. Kassebaum NJ, Bernabé E, Dahiya M, et al. Global burden of severe periodontitis in 1990-2010: a systematic review and meta-regression. J Dent Res 2014;93(11): 1045–53.

15. Varela-Centelles P, Diz-Iglesias P, Estany-Gestal A, et al. Periodontitis awareness amongst the general public: a critical systematic review to identify gaps of knowledge. J Periodontol 2016;87(4):403–15.
16. Genco RJ, Borgnakke WS. Risk factors for periodontal disease. Periodontol 2000 2013;62:59–94.
17. Simpson TC, Weldon JC, Worthington HV, et al. Treatment of periodontal disease for glycaemic control in people with diabetes mellitus. Cochrane Database Syst Rev 2015;(11):CD004714.
18. Martens L, De Smet S, Yusof MY, et al. Association between overweight/obesity and periodontal disease in children and adolescents: a systematic review and meta-analysis. Eur Arch Paediatr Dent 2017;18(2):69–82.
19. Dietrich T, Webb I, Stenhouse L, et al. Evidence summary: the relationship between oral and cardiovascular disease. Br Dent J 2017;222(5):381–5.
20. Cullinan MP, Seymour GJ. Periodontal disease and systemic illness: will the evidence ever be enough? Periodontol 2000 2013;62:271–86.
21. Buset SL, Walter C, Friedmann A, et al. Are periodontal diseases really silent? A systematic review of their effect on quality of life. J Clin Periodontol 2016;43(4):333–44.
22. Faggion CM Jr, Cullinan MP, Atieh M. An overview of systematic reviews on the effectiveness of periodontal treatment to improve glycaemic control. J Periodontal Res 2016;51(6):716–25.
23. Iheozor-Ejiofor Z, Middleton P, Esposito M, et al. Treating periodontal disease for preventing adverse birth outcomes in pregnant women. Cochrane Database Syst Rev 2017;(6):CD005297.
24. Nordenram G, Davidson T, Gynther G, et al. Qualitative studies of patients' perceptions of loss of teeth, the edentulous state and prosthetic rehabilitation: a systematic review with meta-synthesis. Acta Odontol Scand 2013;71(3–4):937–51.
25. Loe H, Theilade E, Jensen SB. Experimental gingivitis in man. J Periodontol 1965;36:177–87.
26. Schätzle M, Löe H, Lang NP, et al. The clinical course of chronic periodontitis. J Clin Periodontol 2004;31(12):1122–7.
27. Lang NP, Schätzle MA, Löe H. Gingivitis as a risk factor in periodontal disease. J Clin Periodontol 2009;36(Suppl 10):3–8.
28. Anerud A, Löe H, Boysen H. The natural history and clinical course of calculus formation in man. J Clin Periodontol 1991;18(3):160–70.
29. Hajishengallis G, Lamont RJ. Beyond the red complex and into more complexity: the polymicrobial synergy and dysbiosis (PSD) model of periodontal disease etiology. Mol Oral Microbiol 2012;27(6):409–19.
30. Hajishengallis G, Darveau RP, Curtis MA. The keystone-pathogen hypothesis. Nat Rev Microbiol 2012;10(10):717–25.
31. Slots J. Herpesviral-bacterial interactions in periodontal diseases. Periodontol 2000 2010;52(1):117–40.
32. Li F, Zhu C, Deng FY, et al. Herpesviruses in etiopathogenesis of aggressive periodontitis: a meta-analysis based on case-control studies. PLoS One 2017;12(10):e0186373.
33. Gao Z, Lv J, Wang M. Epstein-Barr virus is associated with periodontal diseases: a meta-analysis based on 21 case-control studies. Medicine (Baltimore) 2017;96(6):e5980.
34. Vieira AR, Albandar JM. Role of genetic factors in the pathogenesis of aggressive periodontitis. Periodontol 2000 2014;65(1):92–106.

35. Larsson L, Castilho RM, Giannobile WV. Epigenetics and its role in periodontal diseases: a state-of-the-art review. J Periodontol 2015;86(4):556–68.
36. Sonnenschein SK, Meyle J. Local inflammatory reactions in patients with diabetes and periodontitis. Periodontol 2000 2015;69(1):221–54.
37. Nociti FH Jr, Casati MZ, Duarte PM. Current perspective of the impact of smoking on the progression and treatment of periodontitis. Periodontol 2000 2015;67(1): 187–210.
38. Lang NP, Tonetti MS. Periodontal risk assessment (PRA) for patients in supportive periodontal therapy (SPT). Oral Health Prev Dent 2003;1(1):7–16.
39. Page RC, Krall EA, Martin J, et al. Validity and accuracy of a risk calculator in predicting periodontal disease. J Am Dent Assoc 2002;133(5):569–76.
40. Lang NP, Suvan JE, Tonetti MS. Risk factor assessment tools for the prevention of periodontitis progression a systematic review. J Clin Periodontol 2015;42(Suppl 16):S59–70.
41. Diehl SR, Kuo F, Hart TC. Interleukin 1 genetic tests provide no support for reduction of preventive dental care. J Am Dent Assoc 2015;146(3):164–73.e4.
42. Nibali L, Zavattini A, Nagata K, et al. Tooth loss in molars with and without furcation involvement - a systematic review and meta-analysis. J Clin Periodontol 2016; 43(2):156–66.
43. Ramseier CA, Suvan JE. Behaviour change counselling for tobacco use cessation and promotion of healthy lifestyles: a systematic review. J Clin Periodontol 2015;42(Suppl 16):S47–58.
44. Giannobile WV, Braun TM, Caplis AK, et al. Patient stratification for preventive care in dentistry. J Dent Res 2013;92(8):694–701.
45. Ioannidis JP. Preventing tooth loss with biannual dental visits and genetic testing: does it work? J Am Dent Assoc 2015;146(3):141–3.
46. Van der Weijden FA, Slot DE. Efficacy of homecare regimens for mechanical plaque removal in managing gingivitis a meta-review. J Clin Periodontol 2015; 42(Suppl 16):S77–91.
47. Schmalz G, Miller M, Schmickler J, et al. Influence of manual and power toothbrushes on clinical and microbiological findings in initial treatment of periodontitis - a randomized clinical study. Am J Dent 2017;30(1):40–6.
48. Yaacob M, Worthington HV, Deacon SA, et al. Powered versus manual toothbrushing for oral health. Cochrane Database Syst Rev 2014;(6):CD002281.
49. Al Makhmari SA, Kaklamanos EG, Athanasiou AE. Short-term and long-term effectiveness of powered toothbrushes in promoting periodontal health during orthodontic treatment: a systematic review and meta-analysis. Am J Orthod Dentofacial Orthop 2017;152(6):753–66.e7.
50. Sälzer S, Slot DE, Van der Weijden FA, et al. Efficacy of inter-dental mechanical plaque control in managing gingivitis–a meta-review. J Clin Periodontol 2015; 42(Suppl 16):S92–105.
51. Drisko CL. Periodontal self-care: evidence-based support. Periodontol 2000 2013;62(1):243–55.
52. Marchesan JT, Morelli T, Moss K, et al. Interdental cleaning is associated with decreased oral disease prevalence. J Dent Res 2018;97(7):773–8.
53. Kotsakis GA, Lian Q, Ioannou AL, et al. A network meta-analysis of interproximal oral hygiene methods in the reduction of clinical indices of inflammation. J Periodontol 2018;89(5):558–70.
54. Haas AN, Wagner TP, Muniz FW, et al. Essential oils-containing mouthwashes for gingivitis and plaque: meta-analyses and meta-regression. J Dent 2016;55:7–15.

55. Araujo MWB, Charles CA, Weinstein RB, et al. Meta-analysis of the effect of an essential oil-containing mouthrinse on gingivitis and plaque. J Am Dent Assoc 2015;146(8):610–22.

56. James P, Worthington HV, Parnell C, et al. Chlorhexidine mouthrinse as an adjunctive treatment for gingival health. Cochrane Database Syst Rev 2017;(3):CD008676.

57. Slot DE, De Geest S, van der Weijden FA, et al. Treatment of oral malodour. Medium-term efficacy of mechanical and/or chemical agents: a systematic review. J Clin Periodontol 2015;42(Suppl 16):S303–16.

58. Matsubara VH, Bandara HM, Ishikawa KH, et al. The role of probiotic bacteria in managing periodontal disease: a systematic review. Expert Rev Anti Infect Ther 2016;14(7):643–55.

59. Martin-Cabezas R, Davideau JL, Tenenbaum H, et al. Clinical efficacy of probiotics as an adjunctive therapy to non-surgical periodontal treatment of chronic periodontitis: a systematic review and meta-analysis. J Clin Periodontol 2016;43(6): 520–30.

60. Gruner D, Paris S, Schwendicke F. Probiotics for managing caries and periodontitis: Systematic review and meta-analysis. J Dent 2016;48:16–25.

61. Tonetti MS, Chapple IL, Jepsen S, et al. Primary and secondary prevention of periodontal and peri-implant diseases: Introduction to, and objectives of the 11th European Workshop on Periodontology consensus conference. J Clin Periodontol 2015;42(Suppl 16):S1–4.

62. Tonetti MS, Eickholz P, Loos BG, et al. Principles in prevention of periodontal diseases: consensus report of group 1 of the 11th European Workshop on Periodontology on effective prevention of periodontal and peri-implant diseases. J Clin Periodontol 2015;42(Suppl 16):S5–11.

63. Sanz M, Bäumer A, Buduneli N, et al. Effect of professional mechanical plaque removal on secondary prevention of periodontitis and the complications of gingival and periodontal preventive measures: consensus report of group 4 of the 11th European Workshop on Periodontology on effective prevention of periodontal and peri-implant diseases. J Clin Periodontol 2015;42(Suppl 16): S214–20.

64. Chapple IL, Van der Weijden F, Doerfer C, et al. Primary prevention of periodontitis: managing gingivitis. J Clin Periodontol 2015;42(Suppl 16):S71–6.

65. Smiley CJ, Tracy SL, Abt E, et al. Systematic review and meta-analysis on the nonsurgical treatment of chronic periodontitis by means of scaling and root planing with or without adjuncts. J Am Dent Assoc 2015;146(7):508–24.e5.

66. Smiley CJ, Tracy SL, Abt E, et al. Evidence-based clinical practice guideline on the nonsurgical treatment of chronic periodontitis by means of scaling and root planing with or without adjuncts. J Am Dent Assoc 2015;146(7):525–35.

67. ADA center for evidence-based dentistry. Nonsurgical treatment of chronic periodontitis clinical practice guidelines. Available at: https://ebd.ada.org/~/media/EBD/Files/ADA_Chairside_Guide_Periodontitis.pdf?la=en. Accessed April 11, 2018.

68. Sgolastra F, Severino M, Gatto R, et al. Effectiveness of diode laser as adjunctive therapy to scaling root planning in the treatment of chronic periodontitis: a meta-analysis. Lasers Med Sci 2013;28(5):1393–402.

69. Sgolastra F, Severino M, Petrucci A, et al. Nd:YAG laser as an adjunctive treatment to nonsurgical periodontal therapy: a meta-analysis. Lasers Med Sci 2014;29(3):887–95.

70. Behdin S, Monje A, Lin GH, et al. Effectiveness of laser application for periodontal surgical therapy: systematic review and meta-analysis. J Periodontol 2015; 86(12):1352–63.

71. Zandbergen D, Slot DE, Niederman R, et al. The concomitant administration of systemic amoxicillin and metronidazole compared to scaling and root planing alone in treating periodontitis: a systematic review. BMC Oral Health 2016;16:27.

72. Keestra JA, Grosjean I, Coucke W, et al. Non-surgical periodontal therapy with systemic antibiotics in patients with untreated aggressive periodontitis: a systematic review and meta-analysis. J Periodontal Res 2015;50(6):689–706.

73. Zhang Z, Zheng Y, Bian X. Clinical effect of azithromycin as an adjunct to nonsurgical treatment of chronic periodontitis: a meta-analysis of randomized controlled clinical trials. J Periodontal Res 2016;51(3):275–83.

74. Buset SL, Zitzmann NU, Weiger R, et al. Non-surgical periodontal therapy supplemented with systemically administered azithromycin: a systematic review of RCTs. Clin Oral Investig 2015;19(8):1763–75.

75. Ramalho VL, Ramalho HJ, Cipullo JP, et al. Comparison of azithromycin and oral hygiene program in the treatment of cyclosporine-induced gingival hyperplasia. Ren Fail 2007;29:265–70.

76. Eberhard J, Jepsen S, Jervøe-Storm PM, et al. Full-mouth treatment modalities (within 24 hours) for chronic periodontitis in adults. Cochrane Database Syst Rev 2015;(4):CD004622.

77. Polak D, Martin C, Sanz-Sánchez I, et al. Are anti-inflammatory agents effective in treating gingivitis as solo or adjunct therapies? A systematic review. J Clin Periodontol 2015;42(Suppl 16):S139–51.

78. Heitz-Mayfield LJ, Lang NP. Surgical and nonsurgical periodontal therapy. Learned and unlearned concepts. Periodontol 2000 2013;62(1):218–31.

79. Mailoa J, Lin GH, Khoshkam V, et al. Long-term effect of four surgical periodontal therapies and one non-surgical therapy: a systematic review and meta-analysis. J Periodontol 2015;86(10):1150–8.

80. Matarasso M, Iorio-Siciliano V, Blasi A, et al. Enamel matrix derivative and bone grafts for periodontal regeneration of intrabony defects. A systematic review and meta-analysis. Clin Oral Investig 2015;19(7):1581–93.

81. Lee CT, Huang HY, Sun TC, et al. Impact of patient compliance on tooth loss during supportive periodontal therapy: a systematic review and meta-analysis. J Dent Res 2015;94(6):777–86.

82. Trombelli L, Franceschetti G, Farina R. Effect of professional mechanical plaque removal performed on a long-term, routine basis in the secondary prevention of periodontitis: a systematic review. J Clin Periodontol 2015;42(Suppl 16):S221–36.

83. Wilder RS, Bray KS. Improving periodontal outcomes: merging clinical and behavioral science. Periodontol 2000 2016;71(1):65–81.

84. Miller PD Jr, McEntire ML, Marlow NM, et al. An evidenced-based scoring index to determine the periodontal prognosis on molars. J Periodontol 2014;85(2): 214–25.

85. Genco RJ, Genco FD. Common risk factors in the management of periodontal and associated systemic diseases: the dental setting and interprofessional collaboration. J Evid Based Dent Pract 2014;14(Suppl):4–16.

86. Fiorini T, Musskopf ML, Oppermann RV, et al. Is there a positive effect of smoking cessation on periodontal health? A systematic review. J Periodontol 2014;85(1): 83–91.

87. Chambrone L, Preshaw PM, Rosa EF, et al. Effects of smoking cessation on the outcomes of non-surgical periodontal therapy: a systematic review and individual patient data meta-analysis. J Clin Periodontol 2013;40(6):607–15.
88. Farooqi OA, Wehler CJ, Gibson G, et al. Appropriate recall interval for periodontal maintenance: a systematic review. J Evid Based Dent Pract 2015; 15(4):171–81.

How Evidence-Based Dentistry Has Shaped the Practice of Oral Medicine

Katherine France, DMD, MBE, Thomas P. Sollecito, DMD, FDS RCSEd*

KEYWORDS

- Oral medicine • Evidence-based dentistry • Evidence-based practice
- Oral potentially malignant disorders • Temporomandibular disorder
- Salivary dysfunction • Antibiotic prophylaxis

KEY POINTS

- The clinical practice of oral medicine requires guidelines formulated from evidence.
- Clinical Practice Guidelines in oral medicine define recommendations based in evidence.
- For areas with less clarity, emerging evidence base will provide the ability to shape future management recommendations.
- Some areas of oral medicine currently contain only limited evidence, based in expert consensus, and require further research.

INTRODUCTION
Evidence-Based Medicine

Evidence-based medicine has existed as a concept for many years, gaining recognition and respect especially in the past few decades. From its first appearance in the literature, the term "evidence-based medicine"[1] quickly gained prominence,[2] inspiring reviews and Clinical Practice Guidelines focused on using available, carefully gathered proof to define recommendations.[3] These works have defined recommendations for and against medications, surgical interventions, management practices, and diagnostic testing modalities, and they have equally focused scientific awareness on areas in which convincing evidence does not yet exist. Of course, evidence-based medicine is fraught with challenges, including the burden of proof required to formulate Clinical Practice Guidelines, the necessarily narrow definitions of success and end points, and the

Disclosure Statement: K. France has nothing to disclose. T.P. Sollecito serves as a consultant for the American Dental Association Council on Scientific Affairs.
Department of Oral Medicine, University of Pennsylvania School of Dental Medicine, 240 South 40th Street, Philadelphia, PA 19104 USA
* Corresponding author.
E-mail address: tps@upenn.edu

inability for such combined statements to appropriately reflect individual patient presentations or outcomes.[4,5]

Evidence-based guidelines, the studies that support them, and reviews of these studies are formulated by a variety of stakeholders, including patients, practicing clinicians, researchers, policy makers, and health care administrators. One major source of this knowledge, and of support for the synthesis of available data, is the Cochrane Collaboration.[6] The Cochrane Collaboration employs dedicated staff to support subject-specific systematic reviews and meta-analyses, and distributes standards to guide the completion of such studies. Their efforts have helped to spread evidence-based medicine and highlighted its importance for all health care practitioners.

In dental medicine, the importance of evidence-based medicine has experienced a parallel evolution. Soon after evidence-based medicine became a recognized term, the concept of "evidence-based dentistry" likewise started to appear in literature.[7] In the past 15 years, this term has also become widely used to refer to dental practice informed by scientific evidence.[8] As they evolve,[9,10] evidence-based dentistry recommendations have recently become increasingly specialty-specific and procedure-specific.[11–13] As in medicine, evidence must be synthesized and disseminated in dental medicine to inform a Clinical Practice Guideline. The increase in available evidence-based guidelines has and will continue to refine and improve the worldwide practice of dentistry.

Oral Medicine

Oral medicine is a subset of dental medicine that has been defined by various sources. These include the American Academy of Oral Medicine,[14] European Association of Oral Medicine,[15] and multiple groups of practicing oral medicine physicians. In the United States, the definition of oral medicine has been proposed as "the discipline of dentistry concerned with the oral health care of medically complex patients, including the diagnosis and primarily nonsurgical treatment and/or management of medically related conditions affecting the oral and maxillofacial region."[16] The worldwide training of practitioners in this emerging field also has been recently defined, suggesting that residency programs focus on competency in the following:

- Diagnosis and primarily nonsurgical management of oral mucosal and salivary gland disorders
- Diagnosis and primarily nonsurgical management of temporomandibular, orofacial pain, and neurosensory disorders
- Management of the medically complex patient.[17,18]

Oral medicine competency in the United States is in line with the training of oral medicine practitioners worldwide,[18] although some variation exists between countries in scope of practice.

Clinical care in oral medicine is available across the United States in many practice settings, including hospitals, medical/dental schools, and private practice clinics. As defined by a recent study, patients are referred for oral medicine evaluation by a wide variety of practitioners, most commonly general dentists.[19] Referrals also come from specialty physicians, including otorhinolaryngologists, hematologists, oncologists, radiation oncologists, rheumatologists, and dermatologists. As a dedicated link between dental and medical care, oral medicine physicians provide thorough medical and dental evaluations to reach an accurate diagnosis and recommend appropriate treatment. Broadly speaking, oral medicine providers are frequently consulted for evaluation, diagnosis, and treatment of oral lesions, salivary gland diseases, facial pain conditions, and care of medically complex patients. Some examples of these conditions are highlighted in **Box 1**.

Treatment recommendations in oral medicine depend on the individual patient presentation, but in many cases consists of medications, behavioral modifications, and/or oral appliance fabrication. Patients may also be referred for medical evaluation

---

Box 1
Conditions evaluated and managed by oral medicine physicians

- Oral mucosal diseases/oral and perioral lesions[20,21]
  - Oral lesions, including erythroplakia, leukoplakia, oral submucosal fibrosis, pigmented lesions, ulcerations, or lesions associated with systemic conditions, including human immunodeficiency virus (HIV) disease
  - Mucosal and perioral growths, such as fibroma, papilloma, hemangioma, seborrheic keratosis, actinic keratosis
  - Ulcerative diseases, including recurrent aphthous stomatitis and Behçet disease
  - Fungal infections, including angular cheilitis, candidiasis, or deep fungal infection (aspergillosis, histoplasmosis, mucormycosis, blastomycosis)
  - Viral infections, including herpetic infections, Coxsackie infections
  - Immune-mediated disorders, including erythema multiforme, oral lichen planus, mucous membrane pemphigoid, pemphigus vulgaris, or systemic lupus erythematosus
  - Granulomatous disease, including orofacial granulomatosis and oral manifestations of systemic granulomatous disease
  - Malignant conditions of the oral cavity
  - Complications following medical treatments, including oral mucositis, oral graft-versus-host disease, osteonecrosis of the jaw

- Salivary gland disease and dysfunction[22]
  - Objective hyposalivation, caused by medications or previous exposure to radiation therapy
  - Reduced salivary flow secondary to systemic diseases, including Sjögren syndrome and other autoimmune diseases
  - Xerostomia, the subjective feeling of oral dryness
  - Sialosis, enlargement of salivary glands
  - Sialoadenitis, including infections of the salivary glands, such as parotitis
  - Sialolithiasis, stones in the salivary glands
  - Enlargement of salivary glands, as can occur in bulimia nervosa
  - Diffuse infiltrative lymphocytosis syndrome in HIV disease
  - Salivary gland malignances

- Facial pain conditions[23]
  - Pain and dysfunction originating from the temporomandibular joint (TMJ) complex including myalgia, myofascial pain, TMJ capsulitis, TMJ arthralgia, and internal derangement of the TMJ
  - Intraoral pain, including pain of odontogenic, periodontal, mucosal, or bone origin
  - Neuropathic pains involving the oral cavity, including glossodynia or burning mouth syndrome
  - Persistent idiopathic facial pain (atypical facial pain)
  - Neuralgias of the orofacial region including trigeminal, auriculotemporal, and glossopharyngeal neuralgias
  - Headache disorders, including tension-type headache, migraine, cluster headache, and rare autonomic cephalgias
  - Pain of intracranial origin
  - Referred pain from other sites or associated structures
  - Pain arising as a complication of mental illness

- Medically complex patient dental care
  - Assessment of patient fitness for dental treatment
  - Provision or modification of appropriate dental treatment to patients with multiple or complex systemic diseases

when an oral cavity finding suggests a systemic disease. For patients with significant medical comorbidities, the role of the oral medicine practitioner also includes consulting with other members of the health care team and advising on the appropriate modifications to dental treatment or timing of treatment.

The importance of evidence-based practice in oral medicine stems directly from the theoretic and practical complexity of the field. The wide variety of conditions encountered in an oral medicine practice, as well as variations in the individual patient presentation and response to treatment, defines the need for careful evaluation and synthesis of practice recommendations to provide appropriate and effective treatment. The remainder of this article presents examples of how evidence related to each practice area of oral medicine has shaped clinical practice. Our examples show how the use of Clinical Practice Guidelines varies by topic and has evolved over time. They include a recently published Clinical Practice Guideline on the detection of potentially malignant oral disorders to show how evidence guides diagnostic practice, a review on treatment of salivary gland dysfunction that illustrates how existing data inform practice and refine additional study, a review of treatment for temporomandibular disorders that highlights the need for definitive diagnostic criteria, and a Clinical Practice Guideline on the use of prophylactic antibiotics in patients with prosthetic joint replacement to show how evidence-based dentistry benefits society. By highlighting existing examples, we also call attention to the need for further evidence-based guidelines to refine all areas of oral medicine practice.

ORAL LESIONS

Oral lesions present a broad and primary focus of oral medicine practices. As exemplified in **Box 1**, oral lesions can take on an almost infinite variety of clinical appearances based on their size, location, color, texture, and number. They may themselves be benign, premalignant, or malignant, and each lesion may provide information about underlying systemic conditions. Distinguishing based on these and other signs, as well as on symptoms and history can provide clues to the diagnosis of these lesions.

Oral lesions are common in the general population. In an early study, it was estimated that 10% of 23,616 patients studied had at least one oral lesion.[24] These lesions ranged from solitary to widespread, from benign to malignant, and included all surfaces of the oral mucosa. Recognition and evaluation of these lesions is an important aspect of dental treatment. Accurate and thorough clinical evaluation and diagnostic testing are required to determine whether a given lesion may represent a potentially cancerous or a cancerous process.

The importance of early and accurate diagnosis of potentially malignant conditions cannot be overstated. Cancers of the oral cavity, 90% of which are squamous cell carcinoma,[25] are estimated by the American Cancer Society to have accounted for 32,670 new cases and 6650 deaths in 2017.[26] These are separated from cancers of the oropharynx, which accounted for approximately 17,000 new cases and 3050 deaths in 2017. The separation between the oral cavity and the oropharynx is defined as the soft palate, tonsillar pillars, and the base of the tongue, with the oral cavity comprising those areas anterior, including the mobile portion of the tongue, and the oropharynx including these borders and structures posterior. Squamous cell carcinoma of the oral cavity has an overall 5-year survival rate of 64.3% in the United States, with the rate dropping to 38.5% in patients who present with distant metastases.[27] A wide body of literature covers the importance of careful screening of patients in general and specialty dental practice by trained providers to ensure early diagnosis and appropriate referral to treatment for all patients with oral lesions to improve these rates.[28–32]

Given the importance of a timely and accurate diagnosis of malignancies, the assessment of potentially malignant oral lesions depends closely on robust evidence. Multiple studies have been completed and synthesized into a few systematic reviews on the use of diagnostic tests and adjuncts for diagnosis of oral lesions, which reinforce the impact of clear evidence-based recommendations.[33–36] Still other studies have discussed the proper approach to lesions found to contain some level of epithelial dysplasia, although consensus on treatment of these lesions has not yet been established.[37] Synthesizing previous recommendations, a recent report from the American Dental Association provided a Clinical Practice Guideline for evaluation of potentially malignant oral lesions.[38]

This guideline reviews the level of evidence supporting various modalities available for evaluation of a potentially malignant oral disorder. The methods reviewed include the histopathological testing of lesions, salivary analysis, and use of adjunctive tests, such as cytologic sampling, oral mucosal staining, autofluorescence, or vital staining for adults with suspicious lesions in the oral cavity. Using available systematic reviews, as well as studies dealing with efficacy of adjunctive testing, the expert panel was able to reach recommendations for the use of these methods, which appear in **Box 2**.

These carefully compiled and clearly explained guidelines can now be used to inform the clinical practice of providers in all specialties who manage these patients.[39,40] The clinical evaluation of these lesions will thus be shaped by evidence on which methods of testing are most reliable.

SALIVARY GLAND DISEASE

The management of salivary gland disease is an area of oral medicine in which existing treatment recommendations are available to guide expert decisions. As noted

---

Box 2

Recommendations on the evaluation of potentially malignant oral disorders (PMDs)

- The panel suggests that for adult patients with a clinically evident oral mucosal lesion considered to be suspicious of a PMD or malignant disorder, or other symptoms, clinicians should perform a biopsy of the lesion or provide immediate referral to a specialist. (Conditional recommendation, low-quality evidence.)

- The panel does not recommend cytologic adjuncts for the evaluation of PMDs among adult patients with clinically evident, seemingly innocuous, or suspicious lesions. Should a patient decline the clinician's recommendation for performing a biopsy of the lesion or referral to a specialist, the clinician can use a cytologic adjunct to provide additional lesion assessment. (Conditional recommendation, low-quality evidence.)

- A positive or atypical cytologic test result reinforces the need for a biopsy or referral. A negative cytologic test result indicates the need for periodic follow-up of the patient. If the clinician detects persistence or progression of the lesion, immediately performing a biopsy of the lesion or referral to a specialist is indicated.

- The panel does not recommend autofluorescence, tissue reflectance, or vital staining adjuncts for the evaluation of PMDs among adult patients with clinically evident, seemingly innocuous, or suspicious lesions. (Conditional recommendation, low-quality evidence to very low quality evidence.)

From Lingen MW, Abt E, Agrawal N, et al. Evidence-based clinical practice guideline for the evaluation of potentially malignant disorders in the oral cavity. J Am Dent Assoc 2017;148(10):720; with permission.

previously, oral medicine practitioners treat both subjective and objective changes to salivary gland function. Those affected by salivary gland complaints represent a large and diverse patient population, with varied presentations stemming from a wide range of causes. Salivary flow rate may be decreased either temporarily or permanently, or may be unchanged while the consistency of saliva is altered.[22] Additionally, salivary glands may change in size, develop infections, or present with other alterations in function. Altered salivary flow is particularly prevalent and difficult to treat. Given the heterogeneous nature of these complaints and the affected population, consensus recommendations are necessary for appropriate management.

Treatment of decreased salivary flow has been informed by recommendations formulated as a result of a systematic review performed during the fourth World Workshop in Oral Medicine.[41] This group synthesized the available evidence through 2005 regarding the treatment of hyposalivation secondary to systemic diseases including Sjögren syndrome. They combined evidence about which diseases cause salivary gland dysfunction and about topical and systemic treatments available. After review, they were able to recommended several agents for treatment (**Box 3**).

Although the evidence available at the time was insufficient to recommend use of topical moisturizers or sialogogues, the experts do recommend trial use of these agents when patient preference and practitioner experience so dictate.

This guideline has materially directed the academic study of salivary gland dysfunction in oral medicine during the past 10 years. As research into salivary gland disease has continued, this guideline has served as an evidence base in many systematic and narrative reviews.[42–47] The included recommendations for research have informed the study of Sjögren syndrome, other causes of xerostomia, and the role that systemic disease plays in salivary changes. In addition, studies have examined prescription and nonprescription treatments for patients with xerostomia and hyposalivation.[48–51] This guideline has shaped both practice and research focused on patients with salivary gland dysfunction. It allows for oral medicine physicians to provide evidence-based recommendations and for patients to receive the most effective care and guide the field in avenues of further research.

Box 3
Recommendations for the treatment of patients with salivary gland dysfunction

The World Workshop in Oral Medicine working group recommends the following:
- The use of pilocarpine for [radiation-induced or Sjögren syndrome (SS)-induced xerostomia]. The recommended dosage is 5 mg orally 3 times a day with titration up to 10 mg. Classification of Recommendation class I, Level of Evidence A.
- Cevimeline 30 mg, 3 times a day orally, is given as a useful treatment for hyposalivation and xerostomia in primary and secondary SS. Classification of Recommendation class I, Level of Evidence A.
- 150 IU interferon lozenges 3 times daily may enhance salivary secretion in patients with primary SS. Classification of Recommendation class IIa, Level of Evidence A.
- Anti–tumor necrosis factor-α agents (infliximab, etanercept) are NOT recommended at this time to treat hyposalivation in patients with SS. Classification of Recommendation class III, Level of Evidence A.
- Findings suggest that rituximab is effective in the treatment of primary SS. Larger [randomized controlled] trials are needed to draw any conclusions about the efficacy of rituximab.

Data from von Bultzingslowen I, Sollecito TP, Fox PC, et al. Salivary dysfunction associated with systemic diseases: systematic review and clinical management recommendations. Oral Surg Oral Med Oral Pathol Oral Radiol Endod 2007;103:S57.e1-15.

FACIAL PAIN

Facial pain may be the most frequent complaint in an oral medicine practice. This broad topic is associated with a wide number of distinct etiologies, including odontogenic pain, temporomandibular joint (TMJ) pain, neuropathy, headache disorders, and systemic conditions that present with facial pain, including giant cell arteritis and cancers of adjacent structures.[52] In these areas, more detailed work is needed based on each specific diagnosis given the heterogeneity of the causes of facial pain. Each associated topic will benefit from focused evidence-based reviews that inform and standardize clinical practice. At this time, literature on these conditions comes mostly from narrative and opinion-based reviews.[53-57] One area in which some evidence base exists is in the pharmacologic treatment of TMJ-associated pains.

To effectively treat temporomandibular disorders (TMDs), the oral medicine provider must first formulate an appropriate diagnosis based on history and thorough examination of all structures in the TMJ complex. Once the cause of the patient's pain or dysfunction is elucidated, modalities of treatment can be considered. The oral medicine provider may use multiple treatments, beginning frequently with pharmacotherapy, manual manipulation, splint therapy, or trigger point injections, and progressing later to surgical management as needed.[58-60] The most commonly used method for managing pain due to an arthrogenous or myogenous TMJ disorder is pharmacotherapy. Numerous medication classes have been used in practice and proposed in the literature to treat these conditions, including nonsteroidal anti-inflammatories, corticosteroids, muscle relaxants, benzodiazepines, antidepressants, anticonvulsants, opioids, and topical formulations of a variety of medications.[61-63] Given the wide variation in both medication class and individual agent, it is clear that synthesis of available evidence is required to direct clinical practice.

Responding to this need, in 2010, Mujakperuo and colleagues[64] partnered with the Cochrane Collaboration to complete a review on the available evidence for pharmacologic treatment of TMJ disorders. They performed a systematic review of available randomized controlled trials in which a pharmacologic agent was used to treat pain coming from any TMJ diagnosis. Studies included were required to involve pharmacologic treatment of adults with moderate to severe pain in the TMJ or masticatory muscles that had lasted for at least 3 months. This pain could be associated with asymmetric or limited movement, as defined by McNeill's 1997 diagnostic criteria for TMD.[65] The studies were not, however, separated based on the source of the pain, and largely included small treatment groups and other methodological flaws. Partially resulting from these limitations, the review found "insufficient evidence to support or not support the effectiveness of the reported drugs for the management of pain due to TMD."[64]

Lack of definitive recommendation notwithstanding, the clear summary of available evidence in this review serves as an important resource for clinicians that manage patients suffering from TMJ disorders. Due to a paucity of evidence, clinicians often use their own clinical experience and scientific reasoning to shape their practice. Certainly, some differences in prescribing practice are also due to variation in individual patient presentation and provider treatment philosophy, and based on evidence from smaller studies or case series. However, the lack of evidence-based consensus may also contribute to the significant variability in prescribing habits.

This review highlights the need for use of refined and widely accepted diagnostic criteria in TMD to allow for direct comparison between studies. For example, the Diagnostic Criteria for Temporomandibular Disorders for Clinical and Research Applications exists to standardize research design.[66] With carefully applied diagnostic criteria, TMDs can be appropriately separated or compared, and future studies can be designed to address gaps in knowledge. This will eventually provide sufficient evidence for a Clinical Practice Guideline on temporomandibular disorders that contains focused treatment recommendations.

MEDICALLY COMPLEX CARE

Dental treatment of medically complex patients is by definition broad, as it requires a thorough assessment of the patient to determine fitness to undergo dental procedures, as well as determination of the necessary modifications, if any, to treatment. This subject matter falls under the purview of oral medicine, given the field's unique position as both a medical and dental discipline. This dual identity means that oral medicine providers possess a thorough understanding of both the nature of dental treatment and the intricacies of a patient's medical condition. Modifying dental care is also a topic that relies on evidence-based recommendation, as patient safety during dental treatment must be carefully protected. Dental care for medically complex patients requires a review of available evidence and creation of Clinical Practice Guidelines to protect societal well-being.

Evidence-based reviews are necessary to inform clinical management of the interplay between medical morbidities and dental care. Many medical conditions have been reviewed in the dental literature over several decades, with investigators addressing what possible complications may arise for these patients during dental treatment and how best to approach their care.[67–71] These include, notably, guidelines for the use of antibiotic prophylaxis before dental treatment for patients at risk of developing bacterial endocarditis,[72–75] and recommendations against the discontinuation of anticoagulation before invasive dental procedures.[76–79]

An area that has received significant attention is the question of whether patients who have previously undergone various surgical procedures require antibiotic prophylaxis before dental treatment.[80–82] Most notably, much study has focused on whether prophylactic antibiotic therapy before dental treatment will lower the risk of prosthetic joint infection in patients who have previously undergone prosthetic joint replacement.

To address this question, the American Dental Association created a definitive evidence-based Clinical Practice Guideline for use of antibiotic prophylaxis in patients with prosthetic joint replacements.[83] This review compiled all available evidence from both dental and orthopedic literature on the incidence and sequelae of prosthetic joint infection after dental treatment. Based on available literature, the expert panel "judged with moderate certainty that there is no association between dental procedures and the occurrence of [prosthetic joint infection]s."[81] Although data were only available relating to infections in prosthetic hip and knee joints, the lack of association between dental treatment and joint infections was judged to be applicable to all joint replacements given the anatomic similarity between joints. With this evidence, the panel opined that "in general, for patients with prosthetic joint implants, prophylactic antibiotics are not recommended prior to dental procedures to prevent prosthetic joint infection."[81]

The findings of this Clinical Practice Guideline, discouraging across-the-board use of prophylactic antibiotics for patients after prosthetic joint replacement, ensures patient safety. In addition, limiting prescriptions of antibiotics benefits both individual patients and the general population by combatting the growing problems of antibiotic resistance. These guidelines have shaped dental practice since their publication. They provide one clear example of the ways in which creation of a Clinical Practice Guideline benefits the practice of dentistry, the care of individual patients, and society at large.

SUMMARY

The field of oral medicine concentrates on patients with oral lesions, mucosal disease, salivary gland dysfunction, facial pain conditions, and complex medical histories. Through treating affected patients and advising on these complex conditions, oral medicine practitioners serve as leaders in dentistry, and their connection to both medicine and dentistry provides oral medicine with a unique perspective on health care and patient well-being. The intricate clinical conditions and patient presentations encountered in oral medicine necessitate that patient care be approached in a clear and organized fashion. Evidence-based Clinical Practice Guidelines provide this clarity by compiling all available scientific evidence and providing recommendations on diagnosis and treatment.

Although much of dentistry, including oral medicine, continues to be informed by provider experience and training, the standards in the field have adapted according to the information available as Clinical Practice Guidelines have been produced. As illustrated here, guidelines produced on a variety of subjects have helped to guide clinical practice in oral medicine. Existing guidelines have limited the prescription of antibiotics by recommending against their use in patients with prosthetic joint replacements. Expert recommendations have also shaped both research and practice in treatment of salivary gland disease. New guidelines on the treatment of PMDs will direct future evaluation of suspicious lesions. In facial pain, existing evidence highlights the need for definitive diagnostic criteria that directs future study. Through this spread of information, general dentistry practice has and will continue to demonstrate improved understanding of difficult patient presentations and appropriate evaluation, management, and referrals. For those areas and subjects currently without clear guidelines, further study and synthesis of information will lead to improved patient care.

REFERENCES

1. Guyatt GH. Evidence-based medicine. ACP J Club 1991;114:A-16.
2. Evidence-Based Medicine Work Group. Evidence-based medicine: a new approach to teaching the practice of medicine. JAMA 1992;268(17):2420–5.
3. Smith R, Rennie D. Evidence-based medicine–an oral history. JAMA 2014;311(4): 365–7.
4. Greenhalgh T, Howick J, Maskrey N, Evidence Based Medicine Renaissance Group. Evidence based medicine: a movement in crisis? Br Med J 2014;348: g3725.
5. Baeten D, van Hagen PM. Use of TNF blockers and other targeted therapies in rare refractory immune-mediated inflammatory diseases: evidence-based or rational? Ann Rheum Dis 2010;69:2067–73.
6. Higgins JPT, Green S, editors. Cochrane handbook for systematic reviews of interventions 4.2.6. 2006. Available at: http://www.cochrane.org/resources/handbook/hbook.htm. Accessed October 6, 2006.
7. Richards D, Lawrence A. Evidence based dentistry. Br Dent J 1995;179(7):270–3.
8. Karimbux NY. Evidence-based dentistry. J Dent Educ 2013;77(2):123.
9. Faggion CM Jr. The development of evidence-based guidelines in dentistry. J Dent Educ 2013;77(2):124–36.
10. Brignardello-Petersen R, Carrasco-Labra A, Glick M, et al. A practical approach to evidence-based dentistry: understanding and applying the principles of EBD. J Am Dent Assoc 2014;145(11):1105–7.

11. Bayne SC, Fitzgerald M. Evidence-based dentistry as it relates to dental materials. Compend Contin Educ Dent 2014;35(1):18–24.
12. Bidra AS. Evidence-based prosthodontics: fundamental considerations, limitations, and guidelines. Dent Clin North Am 2014;58(1):1–17.
13. Tinanoff N, Coll JA, Dhar V, et al. Evidence-based update of pediatric dental restorative procedures: preventive strategies. J Clin Pediatr Dent 2015;39(3): 193–7.
14. American Academy of Oral Medicine. AAOM: representing the discipline of oral medicine. In: The American Academy of Oral Medicine. 2018. Available at: http://www.aaom.com. Accessed March 3, 2018.
15. European Association of Oral Medicine. Objectives. In: About EAOM. 2017. Available at: http://www.eaom.eu/eaom-about/mission-objectives. Accessed March 3, 2018.
16. Sollecito TP, Rogers H, Prescott-Clements L, et al. Oral medicine: defining an emerging specialty in the United States. J Dent Educ 2013;77(4):392–4.
17. Whitney EM, Stoopler E, Brennan MT, et al. Competencies for the new postdoctoral oral medicine graduate in the United States. Oral Surg Oral Med Oral Pathol Oral Radiol 2015;120(3):324–8.
18. Steele JC, Clark HJ, Hong CHL, et al. World workshop on oral medicine VI: an international validation study of clinical competencies for advanced training in oral medicine. Oral Surg Oral Med Oral Pathol Oral Radiol 2015;120(2):143–51.
19. Pinto A, Khalaf M, Miller CS. The practice of oral medicine in the United States in the twenty-first century: an update. Oral Surg Oral Med Oral Pathol Oral Radiol 2015;119(4):408–15.
20. Sollecito TP, Stoopler ET. Clinical approaches to oral mucosal disorders. Dent Clin North Am 2013;57(4):561–718.
21. Sollecito TP, Stoopler ET. Clinical approaches to oral mucosal disorders: part II. Dent Clin North Am 2014;58(2):265–462.
22. Mandel L. Salivary gland disorders. Med Clin North Am 2014;98:1407–49.
23. DeRossi SS, Sirois DA. Orofacial pain. Dent Clin North Am 2013;57(3):383–560.
24. Bouquot JE. Common oral lesions found during a mass screening examination. J Am Dent Assoc 1986;112:50–7.
25. Rhodus NL, Kerr AR, Patel K. Oral cancer: leukoplakia, premalignancy, and squamous cell carcinoma. Dent Clin North Am 2014;58(2):315–40.
26. Siegel RL, Miller KD, Jemal A. Cancer statistics, 2017. CA Cancer J Clin 2017; 67(1):7–30.
27. Howlander N, Noone AM, Krapcho M, et al, editors. SEER cancer statistics review. Bethesda (MD): National Cancer Institute; 2015. Available at: https://seer.cancer.gov/csr/1975_2010/. Accessed March 3, 2018.
28. Adams D. Oral cancer: early diagnosis. Dent Today 2014;33(4):8.
29. Moyer VA, U.S. Preventive Services Task Force. Screening for oral cancer: U.S. Preventive Service Task Force recommendation statement. Ann Intern Med 2014;160(1):55–60.
30. Brocklehurst P, Kujan O, O'Malley LA, et al. Screening programmes for the early detection and prevention of oral cancer. Cochrane Database Syst Rev 2013;(11):CD004150.
31. Fanaras N, Warnakulasuriya S. Oral cancer diagnosis in primary care. Prim Dent J 2016;5(1):64–8.
32. Ogden G, Lewthwaite R, Shepherd SD. Early detection of oral cancer: how do I ensure I don't miss a tumour? Dent Update 2013;40(6):462–5.

33. Macey R, Walsh T, Brocklehurst P, et al. Diagnostic tests for oral cancer and potentially malignant disorders in patients presenting with clinically evidence lesions. Cochrane Database Syst Rev 2015;(5):CD010276.

34. Walsh T, Liu JL, Brocklehurst P, et al. Clinical assessment to screen for the detection of oral cavity cancer and potentially malignant disorders in apparently healthy adults. Cochrane Database Syst Rev 2013;(11):CD010173.

35. Gualtero DF, Suarez Castillo A. Biomarkers in saliva for the detection of oral squamous cell carcinoma and their potential use for early diagnosis: a systematic review. Acta Odontol Scand 2016;74(3):170–7.

36. Stuani VT, Rubira CM, Sant'Ana AC, et al. Salivary biomarkers as tools for oral squamous cell carcinoma diagnosis: a systematic review. Head Neck 2017; 39(4):797–811.

37. Mehanna HM, Rattay T, Smith J, et al. Treatment and follow-up of oral dysplasia–a systematic review and meta-analysis. Head Neck 2009;31(12):1600–9.

38. Lingen MW, Abt E, Agrawal N, et al. Evidence-based clinical practice guideline for the evaluation of potentially malignant disorders in the oral cavity. J Am Dent Assoc 2017;148(10):712–27.

39. Nadeau C, Kerr AR. Evaluation and management of oral potentially malignant disorders. Dent Clin North Am 2018;62(1):1–27.

40. Lingen M, Tampi M, Urquhart O, et al. Adjuncts for the evaluation of potentially malignant disorders in the oral cavity: diagnostic test accuracy systematic review and meta-analysis. J Am Dent Assoc 2017;148(11):797–813.

41. von Bultzingslowen I, Sollecito TP, Fox PC, et al. Salivary dysfunction associated with systemic diseases: systematic review and clinical management recommendations. Oral Surg Oral Med Oral Pathol Oral Radiol Endod 2007;103:S57.e1-15.

42. Hanchanale S, Adkinson L, Daniel S, et al. Systematic literature review: xerostomia in advanced cancer patients. Support Care Cancer 2014;23(3):881–8.

43. Gonzalez S, Sung H, Sepulveda D, et al. Oral manifestations and their treatment in Sjogren's syndrome. Oral Dis 2014;20(2):153–61.

44. Margaix-Muñoz M, Bagan JV, Poveda R, et al. Sjogren's syndrome of the oral cavity. Review and update. Med Oral Patol Oral Cir Bucal 2009;14(7):e325–30.

45. Napeñas JJ, Brennan MT, Fox PC. Diagnosis and treatment of xerostomia (dry mouth). Odontology 2009;97(2):76–83.

46. Karteek P, Ranjith A, Kethireddy S. Sjogren's syndrome: a review of clinical features, diagnosis and treatments available. Int J Pharm Sci Res 2010;5(1):93–9.

47. Wolff A, Fox PC, Porter S, et al. Established and novel approaches for the management of hyposalivation and xerostomia. Curr Pharm Des 2012;18(34): 5515–21.

48. Chamani G, Shakibi MR, Zarei MR, et al. Assessment of relationship between xerostomia and oral health-related quality of life in patients with rheumatoid arthritis. Oral Dis 2017;23(8):1162–7.

49. Morales-Bozo I, Ortega-Pinto A, Rojas Alcayaga G, et al. Evaluation of the effectiveness of chamomile (*Matricaria chamomilla*) and linseed (*Linum usitatissimum*) saliva substitute in the relief of xerostomia in elders. Gerodontology 2017;34(1): 42–8.

50. Matczuk J, Zalewska A, Łukaszuk B, et al. Effect of streptozotocin-induced diabetes on lipids metabolism in the salivary glands. Prostaglandins Other Lipid Mediat 2016;126(1):9–15.

51. Dalodom S, Lam-ubol A, Jeanmaneechotechai S. Influence of oral moisturizing jelly as a saliva substitute for the relief of xerostomia in elderly patients with hypertension and diabetes mellitus. Geriatr Nurs 2016;37(2):101–9.

52. Zakrzewska JM. Differential diagnosis of facial pain and guidelines for management. Br J Anaesth 2013;111(1):95–104.
53. Graff-Radford S, Gordon R, Ganal J, et al. Trigeminal neuralgia and facial pain imaging. Curr Pain Headache Rep 2015;19(6):19.
54. Silvestre FJ, Silvestre-Rangil J, Lopez-Jornet P. Burning mouth syndrome: a review and update. Rev Neurol 2015;60(10):457–63.
55. DeRossi SS. Orofacial pain: a primer. Dent Clin North Am 2013;57(3):383–92.
56. Forssell H, Jääskeläinen S, List T, et al. An update on pathophysiological mechanisms related to idiopathic orofacial pain conditions with implications for management. J Oral Rehabil 2015;42(4):300–22.
57. Balasubramaniam R, Klasser GD. Orofacial pain syndromes: evaluation and management. Med Clin North Am 2014;98:1385–405.
58. DeRossi SS, Greenberg MG, Liu F, et al. Temporomandibular disorders: evaluation and management. Med Clin North Am 2014;98:1353–84.
59. Liu F, Steinkeler A. Epidemiology, diagnosis, and treatment of temporomandibular disorders. Dent Clin North Am 2013;57:465–79.
60. deSouza RF, Lovato da Silva CH, Nasser M, et al. Interventions for the management of temporomandibular joint osteoarthritis. Cochrane Database Syst Rev 2012;(4):CD007261.
61. Hersh EV, Balasubramiam R, Pinto A. Pharmacologic management of temporomandibular disorders. Oral Maxillofacial Surg Clin N Am 2008;20:197–210.
62. Dym H, Bowler D, Zeidan J. Pharmacologic treatment for temporomandibular disorders. Dent Clin North Am 2016;60:367–79.
63. Wieckiewicz M, Boening K, Wiland P, et al. Reported concepts for the treatment modalities and pain management of temporomandibular disorders. J Headache Pain 2015;16:106.
64. Mujakperuo HR, Watson M, Morrison R, et al. Pharmacological interventions for pain in patients with temporomandibular disorders. Cochrane Database Syst Rev 2010;(10):CD004715.
65. McNeill C. History and evolution of TMD concepts. Oral Surg Oral Med Oral Pathol Oral Radiol Endod 1997;83:51–60.
66. Schiffman E, Ohrbach R, Truelove E, et al. Diagnostic criteria for temporomandibular disorders (DC/TMD) for clinical and research applications: recommendations of the international RDC/TMD consortium network and orofacial pain special interest group. J Oral Facial Pain Headache 2014;28(1):6–27.
67. Parnell AG. The medically compromised patient. Int Dent J 1986;36(2):77–82.
68. Napeñas JJ, Kujan O, Arduino PG, et al. World workshop on oral medicine VI: controversies regarding dental management of medically complex patients: assessment of current recommendations. Oral Surg Oral Med Oral Pathol Oral Radiol 2015;120(2):207–26.
69. Little JW, Miller CS, Rhodus NL. Little and Falace's dental management of the medically compromised patient. 9th edition. St. Louis (MO): Elselvier; 2017.
70. Renton T, Woolcombe S, Taylor T, et al. Oral surgery: part 1. Introduction and the management of the medically compromised patient. Br Dent J 2013;215(5):213–23.
71. Hupp WS, Firriolo FJ, DeRossi SS. Laboratory evaluation of chronic medical conditions for dental treatment: part III. Hematology. Compend Contin Educ Dent 2011;32(7):10–8.
72. Glenny AM, Oliver R, Roberts GJ, et al. Antibiotics for the prophylaxis of bacterial endocarditis in dentistry. Cochrane Database Syst Rev 2013;(10):CD003813.

73. Wilson W, Taubert KA, Gewitz M, et al. Prevention of infective endocarditis: guidelines from the American Heart Association: a guideline from the American Heart Association Rheumatic Fever, Endocarditis, and Kawasaki Disease Committee, Council on Cardiovascular Disease in the Young, and the Council on Clinical Cardiology, Council on Cardiovascular Surgery and Anesthesia, and the quality of care and outcomes research interdisciplinary working group. Circulation 2007; 116(15):1736–54.

74. Wilson W, Taubert KA, Gewitz M, et al. Prevention of infective endocarditis: guidelines from the American Heart Association: a guideline from the American Heart Association Rheumatic Fever, Endocarditis and Kawasaki Disease Committee, Council on Cardiovascular Disease in the Young, and the Council on Clinical Cardiology, Council on Cardiovascular Surgery and Anesthesia, and the quality of care and outcomes research interdisciplinary working group. J Am Dent Assoc 2008;139(Suppl):3S–24S.

75. Nishimura RA, Otto CM, Bonow RO, et al. 2017 AHA/ACC focused update of the 2014 AHA/ACC guideline for the management of patients with valvular heart disease: a report of the American College of Cardiology/American Heart Association Task Force on clinical practice guidelines. Circulation 2017;135:e1159–95.

76. Wahl MJ, Pinto A, Kilham J, et al. Dental surgery in anticoagulated patients–stop the interruption. Oral Surg Oral Med Oral Pathol Oral Radiol 2015;119(2):136–57.

77. Wahl MJ, Miller CS, Rhodus NL, et al. Anticoagulants are dental friendly. Oral Surg Oral Med Oral Pathol Oral Radiol 2018;125(2):103–6.

78. Lanau N, Mareque J, Giner L, et al. Direct oral anticoagulants and its implications in dentistry: a review of literature. J Clin Exp Dent 2017;9(11):e1346–54.

79. Doganay O, Atalay B, Karadağ E, et al. Bleeding frequency of patients taking ticagrelor, aspirin, clopidogrel, and dual anti platelet therapy after tooth extraction and minor oral surgery. J Am Dent Assoc 2018;149(2):132–8.

80. Hussein H, Brown RS. Risk-benefit assessment for antibiotic prophylaxis in asplenic dental patients. Gen Dent 2016;64(4):62–5.

81. Stoopler ET, Sia YW, Kuperstein AS. Do patients with solid organ transplants or breast implants require antibiotic prophylaxis before dental treatment? J Can Dent Assoc 2012;78:c5.

82. Holland B, Kohler T. Minimizing penile implant infection: a literature review of patient and surgical factors. Curr Urol Rep 2015;16(12):81.

83. Sollecito TP, Abt E, Lockhart PB, et al. The use of prophylactic antibiotics prior to dental procedures in patients with prosthetic joints. J Am Dent Assoc 2015; 146(1):11–6.

Teaching Evidence-Based Practice

Considerations for Dental Education

Robert J. Weyant, MS, DMD, DrPH

KEYWORDS

- Evidence-based dentistry • Dental education • Evidence-based practice

KEY POINTS

- The benefits of providing dentists with evidence-based training are improvements in the quality of patient care.
- The outcomes of evidence-based training on learning and behavior vary based on the type of educational programs used.
- Educational research suggests that integrating didactic with clinical educational programs is important in developing sustained improvements in the use of evidence in clinical practice.
- Contextual or cultural barriers to adopting evidence must be addressed for successful implementation of new evidence.

INTRODUCTION
Statement of the Problem

The problems that occur when high-quality evidence fails to reach routine clinical practice was clearly identified by the Institute of Medicine's review of the US health care system.[1] They identified 3 concerns, which they classified as follows. First, they reported an overuse of treatments that were known to provide no patient benefit. Second, they reported an underuse of treatment know to provide benefit. Finally, they described a misuse of treatment such that care was misapplied to such an extent that patients failed to benefit fully from treatment. This characterization was referred to as the "know–do gap," describing the difference between what is known to work in the way of beneficial treatment and what is actually done in routine patient care.

The attempt to remedy this problem was, in large part, the motivation behind the development of evidence-based practice (EBP) efforts in medicine and other health care professions that evolved from work at McMaster University in the 1990s.[2]

Disclosure Statement: The author has nothing to disclose.
University of Pittsburgh School of Dental Medicine, 3501 Terrace Street, Pittsburgh, PA 15213, USA
E-mail address: Rjw1@pitt.edu

Dent Clin N Am 63 (2019) 97–117
https://doi.org/10.1016/j.cden.2018.08.010
0011-8532/19/© 2018 Elsevier Inc. All rights reserved.

The Sicily Statement, a consensus statement from 2005 on EBP, reads: "All health care professionals need to understand the principles of EBP, recognize EBP in action, implement evidence-based policies, and have a critical attitude to their own practice and to evidence."[3] Dawes and colleagues[3] go on to define EBP and describe a curriculum required to practice in an evidence-based way. To accomplish this, they adopted the 5-step model first described by Cook and colleagues,[4] which is presented in **Table 1**.

These steps have become the foundation for practicing and teaching EBP and are the core of contemporary EBP curricula in health professional schools. This article presents an introduction to current EBP teaching issues and strategies that build on this

Table 1
The 5-step model of evidence-based practice as described by Dawes and colleagues[3] with additional competencies as provided by Young and colleagues[5] (and Rosenberg and colleagues[6])

Sicily Statement[3]	Young and colleagues[5] [Rosenberg and Donald[6]]
Step 1: Translation of uncertainty to an answerable question	ASK: Identify knowledge gaps; Ask focused questions. [Requires knowledge to construct a question using the PICO mnemonic.]
Step 2: Systematic retrieval of best evidence available	ACCESS: Design search strategies; Identify appropriate databases: search effectively and efficiently. [Requires the acquisition and application of literature searching skills across a variety of databases.]
Step 3: Critical appraisal of evidence for validity, clinical relevance, and applicability	APPRAISE: Appraise research for validity, reliability, and applicability; Interpret research findings and translate outcomes into meaningful summary statistics. [Requires a certain level of expertise in epidemiology and biostatistics.]
Step 4: Application of results in practice.	APPLY: Know the approach to assess applicability and generalizability of research findings in clinical practice; evidence-informed decision making. [Requires an ability to synthesize and communicate the results to relevant parties (that is, other health professionals, patients).]
Step 5: Evaluation of performance	AUDIT: Be familiar with the approach to monitor and evaluate practice. [Requires the health professional to evaluate the EBP process and assess its impact within the clinical context in which it was implemented.]

Enabling competencies (Young[5]):
• Biostatistics
• Epidemiology
• Searching electronic databases
• Philosophy of critical enquiry

PICO stands for P, patient, problem or population; I, intervention; C, comparison, control, or comparator; O, outcome.

5-step model. Where available in the literature, evaluation of EBP teaching effectiveness is reviewed. The evaluative literature in this area has grown substantially in recent years, but the majority of the literature continues to come from health care fields outside of dentistry. Thus, one must extrapolate from research done within other health professions, principally medicine and nursing, with the hope that similar findings will apply within dentistry. Additionally, it needs to be noted that this article is not a systematic review of EBP teaching methods. Neither is this a "how to" guide for creating an EBP curriculum, because any curriculum will need to be uniquely adapted based on local conditions, type of student, goals, budget, and other resources. Rather, this article is an introduction to the most salient issues that need to be considered when attempting to construct an EBP curriculum.

GOAL OF TEACHING EVIDENCE-BASED PRACTICE

The motivation for teaching EBP is the assumption that. through the use of high-quality clinically relevant evidence, clinicians will make rational clinical decisions that optimally improve patient health outcomes. To achieve that goal in a sustainable way, clinicians must be able to answer patient care–relevant clinical questions efficiently, which means that they must be able rapidly to retrieve evidence and assess its quality and relevance to their patients. The selection and application of relevant evidence to clinical decision making is understood to proceed most effectively through the use of these widely accepted 5 steps, each step requiring skill that must be learned through formal training programs. This skill development forms the basis for initial EBP educational efforts.

Beyond the 5-step process, effective EBP incorporates the concepts of clinical expertise and patient preferences. Clinical expertise refers to the ability of a health care provider to appropriately translate research findings into clinical care decisions as it applies to an individual patient. Without thoughtful consideration of the clinical status of a patient, the application of research evidence can easily be misapplied. The reason for this is that the clinical research that underlies EBP is typically based on either clinical or epidemiologic studies of populations of patients, with the outcomes of the study being expressed as population parameters such as a group mean response to therapy or other values that convey the likelihood of a given clinical outcome.

In the absence of additional clinical or other relevant information about a given patient, these population-derived values may be considered as the best bet for predicting an individual patient's outcome. However, there are always known and unknown factors that will alter an individual's response to treatment. Skilled clinicians understand this and adapt their application of scientific evidence to the unique circumstances of individual patients.

Patient preferences provide the basis for the ultimate decisions around treatment choices. As such, it is the responsibility of the health care provider to be able to explain the benefits and possible harms of alternative treatment options in an understandable way to each patient. This process also requires a thorough understanding of the relevant evidence as well as skill in communicating with patients (step 4). Communicating scientific information to patients in an understandable way has not be well-studied and tends often to be overlooked in EBP training. This area should not be overlooked in designing EBP educational interventions, especially with novice students, and practical exercises that develop students' abilities in this area should be included in a comprehensive EBP curriculum.

In short, EBP boils down to using valid clinical reasoning informed by current best evidence from high-quality clinical research to recommend personalized approaches to patient care. Such evidence, to be useful for clinical practice, must be readily accessible and understandable to a busy clinician. The skill set required to efficiently find relevant clinical information, determine its validity, and apply that evidence in the care of a given patient is not unusually daunting; nevertheless, it must be learned. Thus, it is appropriate to think of EBP as a set of discrete clinical skills that require training and practice such that they become an ongoing part of routine patient care. The importance of EBP skill to clinical practice is underscored by Glasziou and colleagues,[7] when they affirm that "the search engine is now as essential as the stethoscope" for effective clinical practice.

A chief goal of teaching EBP skills, therefore, is to encourage clinicians to have the confidence and ability to be their own knowledge producers. That concept means that they should be able, on their own, to find and absorb the current best evidence when it is needed for patient care and have the clinical skills to appropriately apply that evidence with individual patients. This should be the overarching goal of EBP teaching. Once mastered, these skills decrease the need to seek out (and pay for) continuing education courses or rely on anecdotal advice from colleagues. Herein, we examine this skill set and how teaching it to dentists can best be accomplished.

A PARADIGM SHIFT IN ACCESSING INFORMATION

Professionals generally understand their obligation to be up to date on current approaches to care. They also understand that new products and approaches to care occur frequently; that patients have access to vast amounts of information online, leading them to ask challenging questions; and that research is continually being published offering new information and critiques of even well-established treatments. In the best case, this leads to clinicians being curious and to routinely seeking answers to questions about what changes have occurred recently that could lead to improved patient care. In the worst case, the thousands of clinical research articles published each year (both high quality and not so high quality) leads to information overload and results in a sense of frustration over the inability to remain well-informed of current clinical developments. Professions and their regulators (eg, state licensing boards, hospital quality management and improvement committees) endeavor to ensure that practitioners make some effort to remain up to date through the use of policy mechanisms, such as mandatory continuing education. But these policies are at best minimal requirements for keeping current with best practices.

Clearly, all health care professionals use evidence in clinical practice. Concern arises primarily when that evidence is outdated, inaccurate, or highly biased and, thus, contributes to less than optimal decision making. Moreover, expanding one's clinical knowledge base, particularly when that is done through reliance on passive, external training (eg, attending continuing education courses), requires the investment of substantial time and resources, often only leading to minimally acceptable compliance with licensure requirements. Moreover, there are often at best negligible quality filters used to ensure that the information delivered through continuing education courses is valid, unbiased, and comports with current scientific knowledge.

The 5-step model originally developed at McMaster University in the 1990s was designed to supplement traditional educational approaches for keeping up to date by taking advantage of changes in technology that were rapidly occurring.[2] Several important changes were ongoing in the 1990s that allowed a reconceptualization of how evidence could be accessed and used in clinical practice. This period saw the

World Wide Web go live globally and in so doing provide the necessary vehicle for rapid dissemination of scientific information over the Internet. In concert with that were advances in online storage of scientific information (eg, Medline) and the ability to efficiently search for information within these massive databases (eg, PubMed) using desktop computers. Capitalizing on these changes, the McMaster group effectively changed the paradigm of how evidence should be used in clinical practice. Rather than relying on random reading of journal articles or attending a continuing education course, it was now possible, in real time, to access highly relevant clinical evidence when and where it was needed in support of patient care decisions. This "just-in-time" approach relieved the burden of information overload and made each clinician his or her personal knowledge producers.

Teaching strategies aimed at improving health professionals' knowledge, attitudes, and skills related to EBP have been evolving since the introduction of the concept of evidence-based medicine by Guyatt and colleagues[2] in 1992. In the United States, accreditation standards associated with the teaching of EBP have resulted in all health care professional schools offering a curriculum in EBP, with the Sicily Statement 5-step model guiding most EBP curricula. These skills are considered essential to allow a clinician to practice in an evidence-based manner.[3] The clinician who has mastered these skills will be able to quickly access valid and relevant evidence, interpret its relevance to their patients, and thus have an objective basis for clinical decision making.

Educational interventions leading to mastery of these skills, along with formal training in critical thinking and statistical reasoning, were a huge advance in creating scientifically literate clinicians. Once basic skills are learned, however, the challenge remains in establishing their application during routine clinical practice. Hurd[8] claims that, when clinicians are comfortable using the scientific literature and it is a routine part of their practice, they move away from passive dependence on the ideas of others and become critical thinkers capable of creating their own new knowledge.

However, after several decades of using this model of EBP training in health professional schools, it is now understood that achieving competency in the 5-step model alone is rarely sufficient to lead to the desired clinical behavioral outcomes where clinicians routinely and rationally apply new evidence in support of patient care. This well-documented resistance to changes in clinician behavior as it relates to patient care must be addressed as part of a comprehensive EBP educational intervention. To accomplish this requires that both the individual and contextual barriers that prevent implementation of new evidence must be overcome. We are now beginning to understand what those barriers are and to develop teaching methods that can aid clinicians in overcoming them.

WHERE DO CLINICIANS TYPICALLY GET INFORMATION?

Research suggests at present that we are failing in creating competent personal knowledge producers and effective evidence-based practitioners. Across health professionals, there is a lack of willingness to search for and understand evidence. It can be instructive to examine what evidence sources are preferred by various health care professionals. Physicians reportedly rely on guidelines, discussion with colleagues, expert consultants (eg, continuing medical education providers), and the pharmaceutical industry as their preferred information sources.[9] Similar results were found among practicing nurses. Dentists report difficulty in applying information from research journal articles, literature searches, and clinical practice guidelines to clinical practice,[10] preferring the more personalized reliance on colleagues and recognized experts (eg, continuing education courses),[11] where evidence is packaged and sold in concise ways that often satisfy the continuing education requirements of licensing boards. Dental students have been shown to prefer seeking information most frequently from colleagues, the Internet (excluding Cochrane Database of Systematic Reviews), and textbooks.[12]

It is worth stating that no source of clinical evidence is inherently inappropriate to inform clinical practice. What needs to be understood is that evidence sources vary in their relevance and validity in answering specific clinical care questions. Systematic reviews are one of the best sources for evidence on comparative treatment efficacy. Clinical practice guidelines play an important role in the dissemination of best practices for clearly specified patient types. Seeking advice from colleagues can be effective ways to gain insight regarding clinical techniques or how to manage unanticipated outcomes.

However, across all health professions, there is a general resistance to seeking out clinical evidence from searching and reading the clinical literature as a means to answer clinical questions. As a result, contrary to what would be hoped—namely, that clinicians personally seek out and implement high-quality evidence as the norm in daily practice—the majority of physicians, nurses, and other health care professionals do not consistently engage in EBP.[13–16]

WHAT ARE THE BARRIERS TO ACCESSING AND USING HIGH-QUALITY EVIDENCE?

Glasgow and colleagues[17] make the case that effective implementation of evidence into routine practice requires attention to both individual provider factors (eg, knowledge, skill, attitudes related to EBP) and broader contextual factors (eg, organizational culture and leadership). Individual knowledge and attitudinal barriers are a significant problem that seem to be related to a lack of understanding of how clinical research is done and how it can inform clinical practice. When asked about their use of the scientific literature, dentists report a distrust or skepticism of evidence-based resources such as systematic reviews and clinical practice guidelines, doubting their validity and the authority of the sources.[18] Hence, using evidence sources believed to be invalid can lead dentists to fear criticism from colleagues or concern over moving beyond a perceived standard of practice.

Structural factors related to the nature of clinical practice create a context for care delivery that reinforces the status quo and is understood to prevent behavior change. Factors commonly reported as barriers to implementing evidence-based changes in clinical care include busy clinic schedules, a potential for the loss of revenue when practice patterns change, workflow inertia, and poor access to high-quality online evidence resources. Large, multiprovider practices suffer from additional organizational barriers (eg, leadership, safety culture, organizational learning, teamwork, and communication issues) that also prevent behavior change.[19]

The lack of easy access to much of the high-quality clinical literature has led Isham[18] to conclude that current evidence dissemination systems and networks aimed at dentists are themselves a major barrier to accessing evidence and contribute to dentists' preference for face-to-face communication, despite the availability of large quantities of quality information online.

Finally, knowledge barriers related to educational deficits can result in clinicians not having the necessary understanding and skill to efficiently search for and apply high-quality evidence in clinical practice.[20] Isham and colleagues[18] identified a lack of knowledge related to using technology (computers, tablets, search engines, etc) as a particular problem among dentists. Additionally, dentists report an inability to synthesize scientific information for clinical applications, an ability that depends on specific critical thinking skills related to scientific and probabilistic reasoning that is not commonly taught in dental schools.

EDUCATIONAL APPROACHES

Perceiving value in a task has been found to support effective learning.[21] Accomplishing that for the EBP material in the dental curriculum can be challenging. Learning the technical or procedural skills (ie, operative or surgical skills) required to perform routine clinical dentistry rightly consumes much of the curricular time as well as students' attention during dental training. These skills are essential and challenging and take time to master. Training students in these clinical skills typically is done through an apprenticeship model, where one practices clinical procedures under the watchful mentorship of clinical faculty members. This learning approach is necessary to safely develop clinical skills, but it can also reinforce students' reliance on authority and focuses the student on the procedures that must be mastered rather than the underlying rationale for when it is appropriate to perform those procedures.[22] The naïve student presumes that authority figures like teachers and experienced clinicians will always provide the right answer to clinical questions, which can undermine in students' minds the relevance of reading research or looking for evidence beyond that provided by the clinical mentors.

Overcoming this dependent learning style is one of the first challenges in teaching EBP to dental students. The importance of developing critical thinking and EBP skills early in the curriculum is, thus, important in providing a learning framework that emphasizes independent, self-learning that will serve the students throughout their professional training and beyond. Providing a strong rationale for why EBP is being taught is thus important. Five areas are suggested as part developing a strong rationale for teaching EBP.

Change Is Not Only Inevitable, It Is Desirable

It is often unclear to the novice student (eg, the first-year dental student) that the knowledge base of the profession changes continually. The novice student's limited perspective on the changing nature of professional practice can lead to a sense that once they learn what is offered in the first professional curriculum, they should be set for life for professional practice. This thinking leads to a reliance on authority figures like teachers and experienced clinicians as the sole source of relevant clinical information and a simultaneous discounting of the value of clinical research.[23] Moreover, the actual approach to teaching used in most dental schools—that is, a reliance on a lecture format—reinforces this thinking. Instilling in students the concept that professional knowledge changes constantly and that it is a professional responsibility to keep up to date on those changes after one leaves their initial training program is an important concept that needs to be introduced early in the curriculum and strongly reinforced in EBP teaching.

Critical Thinking

A second skill lacking in most novice students is relevant critical thinking ability. Algen[23] characterizes clinical practice as uncertain, ambiguous, and constantly changing. Effectively navigating the information needs of clinical practice depends on critical thinking and reasoning. Critical thinking encompasses many domains, but the ones central to EBP teaching are focused on sound judgements related to the validity of research findings and its relevance to patient care. Willignham[24] identifies 3 domains of critical thinking: reasoning, making judgements and decisions, and problem solving. When effective, Willingham says that critical thinking leads to desired outcomes, such as seeing all sides of an argument, accepting new evidence when it disconfirms to your existing ideas, reasoning objectively rather than from passion, and other important traits that improve problem solving. Moreover, critical thinking is also self-directed, meaning that it empowers the individual to seek solutions rather than rely on others for motivation or guidance. Thus, the ability to think critically is foundational for effective EBP because it provides the foundation upon which the application of evidence to clinical practice depends.[25]

Scientific Reasoning

Beyond the general critical thinking qualities described elsewhere in this article, there is an EBP subdomain that Zimmerman[26] refers to as scientific reasoning. This notion implies the third concept required for students, namely, to understand and accept evidence derived from clinical research, which requires a solid foundation in interpreting clinical research studies. Students arrive for clinical training from a variety of backgrounds. Although most come with some sort of science background, it cannot be assumed that their prior training has prepared them for the specific type of scientific reasoning required to understand clinical research and apply it to patient care. Unlike many areas of science, clinical research relies on probabilistic arguments to support conclusions about causal relationships. Windish and colleagues[27] found a lack of knowledge in biostatistics sufficient to interpret many of the results in published clinical research among medical residents. Individuals who understand conditional probabilities and statistical reasoning will more quickly grasp why some clinical research designs are stronger than others in managing bias and why causal arguments in biomedicine are rarely conclusive.

Straub-Morarend and colleagues[12] found low levels of self-confidence among dental students in being able to critically appraise relevant clinical literature. They attributed this in part to students' reported difficulty with statistical concepts and urged more statistical instruction in the predoctoral dental curriculum. Ensuring that learners understand statistical reasoning and probabilities should make it clearer why research study quality depends on methodologic issues, such as the use of control groups, sample size, management of confounding, and the use of statistics to quantify the role of chance. This foundation should include a clear understanding of the strengths and weaknesses of the clinical research designs and what information can be obtained from each.

Hurd[8] frames the goal of teaching scientific reasoning as creating clinicians who are able to distinguish:

- Facts from propaganda (advertisement),
- Probability from certainty,
- Data from assertions,
- Rational belief from superstitions, and
- Science from folklore.

Active Knowledge Acquisition

Conceptualizing EBP as an ongoing clinical activity is important. As highlighted elsewhere in this article, passive dependence on others for new knowledge is ineffective and will become a major barrier to keeping up to date once students leave training. The notion that students must be their own knowledge creators and actively pursue personal knowledge deficits must be emphasized as essential for maintaining current clinical skills and practicing in an ethical manner.

Willingness to Change

Being willing to change one's views and approach to clinical practice in light of new high-quality evidence is perhaps the most challenging skill to teach. The understanding that change in knowledge occurs continually and that it is the responsibility of every health care provider to actively participate in the process of keeping up to date, with an emphasis that changing practice in light of new evidence, is laudable. The challenge lies in the fact that behavior change is bound up in a complex set of personality features and the degree to which one can engage in probabilistic reasoning. For example, presenting a clinician with new evidence that negates prior practice behavior can lead to cognitive dissonance and will often result in denial of the validity of the new evidence.[28] Nevertheless, revising one's behavior in the light of new evidence is clearly an essential skill for effective EBP practice. As Glasziou and colleagues[7] say, "Health professionals cannot solely rely on what they were first taught if they want to do the best for their patients. It has repeatedly been shown that clinical performance deteriorates over time."

EVIDENCE-BASED PRACTICE AS A CLINICAL COMPETENCY

Starting with a clear statement of the EBP learning objectives, framed as competency statements, is likely to improve outcomes of educational intervention as this supports both course content and student evaluation.[29,30] Using competencies to guide the development of educational interventions can help to overcome two of the most commonly reported barriers to effective EBP practice—namely, poor knowledge of the process and skill deficits in performing EBP tasks (such as searching) and critical appraisal.[31]

Competency in EBP is often divided into 4 domains: knowledge, attitudes, skills, and behaviors. Basic EBP competencies can be derived from the 5-step EBP model and additional competencies should be included related to critical thinking, statistical reasoning, clinical problem solving, and communication. **Box 1** provides links to 5 sites that list EBP competencies that are available online.

Framing EBP skills and behavior in terms of clinical competencies is important, because it places these qualities directly alongside other clinical skills (eg, operative procedures). The implication is that, to achieve competency, students must repeatedly practice these skills in routine clinical settings and with various faculty members modeling appropriate EBP behavior. The goal is to form in the student's mind a sense that EBP practice is a central part of the culture of clinical dentistry and is primarily focused on improving clinical outcomes for patients.[37]

Box 1
Sources of evidence-based practice competency statements

- Competencies in Evidence Based Practice for Health Professionals.[32]

- The Establishment of Evidence-Based Practice Competencies for Practicing Registered Nurses.[33]

- An approach on defining competency in evidence-based dentistry. A framework of competency development for dentistry based adult learning theory.[34]

- Center for Evidence Based Medicine Core Competencies.[35]

- A simple real-world competency framework for general practice.[36]

Assessing clinical competency is a familiar practice in dental schools and applying this approach to EPB skills and behaviors should follow a similar tactic. Specifically, competency assessments are best done using valid, behavioral focused assessment tools and demonstrated within the context of the comprehensive care of patients. Ideally, assessment should focus on both short- and long-term outcomes. Most evaluative research of the outcomes of EBP educational intervention's focus on measuring relatively short-term changes occurring within weeks after completion of training. There are a large number of assessment tools reported in the literature for this purpose. Shaneyfelt and colleagues[38] identified 104 different instruments, but few had undergone robust psychometric assessed of their validity and reliability. Most assessment instruments measure short-term outcomes, such as improvement in knowledge and skills but fewer focus on changes in student attitudes and behavior. The most

Table 2 EBP skill assessment instruments	
Berlin[39]	A 15-item multiple choice questionnaire. The instrument focuses on epidemiological knowledge and thus only assesses critical appraisal skill (step 3). Very good psychometric properties and ability to discriminate levels of expertise.
Fresno[38]	Two clinical scenarios and open-ended questions aimed at assessing skills and knowledge related to EBP. Assesses broad EBP knowledge across EBP steps 1–4. Very good psychometric properties and ability to discriminate levels of expertise.
Assessing Competency in EBM (ACE)[40]	A 15-item multiple choice questionnaire to assess competence across all key constructs of EBM (steps 1–4). Good psychometric properties and ability to discriminate levels of expertise.
EBP Competence Questionnaire (EBP-COQ)[41]	A 25-item questionnaire, with 3 categories: attitude, knowledge, and skills. Adequate psychometric properties to measure undergraduate student EBP competencies.
The Evidence-Based Practice Attitude Scale (EBPAS)[42]	A 15-item questionnaire. A brief measure of attitudes toward adopting EBP. Good psychometric properties and likely applicable with a variety of health care disciplines.
Evidence-Based Practice Attitude Scale (EBMQ)[43]	An 80-item questionnaire. Reported to be a valid and reliable instrument to assess the knowledge, practice and barriers toward the implementation of EBM among primary care physicians.
Knowledge, Attitudes, Access, and Confidence Evaluation (KACE)[44]	A 35-item questionnaire. A dental focused questionnaire with 4 subscales that assess knowledge, attitudes, searching skills and overall confidence in assessing evidence quality.

Abbreviation: EBP, evidence-based practice.

widely used assessment instruments now in use are listed in **Table 2**. Most assessment instruments focus on steps 1 to 4 (see **Table 1**). Step 5 is more appropriately assessed through direct observation.

The literature describing long-term outcomes assessing the degree to which the training has led to sustained behavior change in patient care is rare. Long-term studies of clinical behavior and its changes are challenging for numerous methodologic reasons. For example, examining long-term changes in behavior in dental school settings is challenging because it may require follow-up after student graduation. Additionally, it would be difficult to identify an appropriate comparison group. Furthermore, instruments designed to measure long-term changes in behavior are not common and can require observation of behavior in clinical settings by trained evaluators. For those who wish to engage in such research, behavior change measures that emphasize valid and objective reasoning leading to appropriate decisions related to patient care should be used (or developed).

Tilson and colleagues[45] have developed key principles and priorities for developing EBP assessment tools, called the Classification Rubric for EBP Assessment Tools in Education (CREATE). The CREATE tool provides an overall assessment framework based on the 5-step model. Attention is given to both formative and summative assessments. The CREATE framework provides examples and guidance in assessing: knowledge, attitudes, skills, behavior, self-efficacy, and reaction to the educational experience. The approach emphasizes the importance and challenges associated with assessing clinician behavior and patient outcomes as part of any comprehensive assessment program.

DEVELOPING AN EFFECTIVE EVIDENCE-BASED PRACTICE CURRICULUM

Structuring the EBP curriculum in a dental school will certainly need to be customized by local conditions and the literature reflects the large variety of educational approaches now in use, ranging from traditional didactic lectures, small group work, self-directed online courses, and mixed methods. Research suggest that all of these teaching strategies have documented ability in the short term to improve knowledge, attitudes, and skills. Research on these various types of educational interventions, however, have failed to demonstrate the superiority of any particular method.[46] However, some general findings can assist in the development of an effective EBP educational program.

Burn and Foley[47] expressed concern over the ongoing reliance of the traditional lecture approach to deliver curricular content, which they believe reinforces passive learning and a dependence on experts (ie, faculty) as the primary source of knowledge. This lack of focus on critical thinking and scientific reasoning renders students with an inability to evaluate and prioritize sources of information based on their validity and value to clinical practice and undercuts efforts to develop independent self-learning, which is the essence of EBP.

An associated concern results when EBP training is delivered in isolation as a stand-alone didactic course. Although an initial introduction to EBP can be accomplished in a dedicated classroom course on EBP, responsibility for reinforcement throughout the entire clinical curriculum must fall broadly on clinical faculty who teach outside of the classroom. Standalone didactic courses have been shown to be ineffective in improving attitudes and behavior related to EBP.[48] The EBP education research literature suggests that the best outcomes are achieved when the EBP educational intervention uses a mixed method integration of didactic learning with application of EBP principles within routine patient care.[49]

Glasziou and colleagues[7] emphasized the importance of building on the initial EBP training through repeated application in everyday clinical work with the gradual addition of more advanced knowledge and critical thinking skills in clinical settings. Importantly, it has been shown that faculty need to model EBP by demonstrating that "discretion in clinical decision making should be informed by evidence, and not by professionals' personal preferences, habitual routines, or opinion-driven decisions based on traditional practices."[50] Implicit in this approach is having a clinical faculty who are well-versed in EBP skills and routinely model these behaviors in the clinic.

Focusing on short-term learning, evidence from several systematic reviews provides guidance in curriculum development. However methodologic heterogeneity across studies makes conclusions challenging. Phillips and colleagues[51] reviewed 61 studies of EBP educational interventions and found substantial inconsistency among studies in reporting of methods and concluded that, based on the current literature, replication with high fidelity of reported EBP educational interventions would not generally be possible. Nevertheless, the characterization of broad domains of educational interventions in current use provides guidance in developing a curriculum. Häggman-Laitila and colleagues[52] suggest organizing educational interventions around 3 themes: principles of EBD and research, the process of EBP, and preparing for change.

PRINCIPLES OF EVIDENCE-BASED PRACTICE AND RESEARCH

Teaching the principles of EBD focuses on improving students' knowledge, attitudes, and skills. This learning is often initially accomplished in the nonclinical settings (eg, classroom). Lecture format courses may be an appropriate method for delivering the first exposure to basic EBP concepts, but, as stated elsewhere in this article, if used as the sole method of delivering EBP education, it can foster a passive and dependent learning style. Additionally, this method fails to expose students to the expected clinical behavior, making it unlikely that students will develop those behaviors and competencies independently. Beyond classroom lectures, various other methods of presenting EBP content have been studied, often with mixed results, depending on the outcomes measured (eg, knowledge, attitude, skill, and behavior).

Problem-based learning is an approach used in some predoctoral curricula and was found to be less effective in EBP knowledge improvement compared with usual teaching approaches (eg, lectures). One reason the authors named for the poor improvements in knowledge was the students' reported lack of understanding of core statistical knowledge, resulting in their inability to understand and discuss the clinical research literature.[53]

The duration of educational interventions varies from short 2-hour interventions to semester-long course. Shorter courses tended to focus on very specific skill development. For example, Gruppen and colleagues[54] used a nonrandomized control group study design and found efficacy from a single, brief (2-hour) instructional intervention on EBM-based techniques for searching Medline for evidence related to a clinical problem provided to the students. Providing a comprehensive educational program delivered in short doses such as this might be desirable in some settings, such as part of a faculty development program or for online training for practicing dentists. These investigators also found that adding a medical librarian to the teaching staff improved outcomes.[55]

Fritsche and colleagues[39] found effectiveness in both knowledge and skills with a 3-day intensive workshop among postgraduate physicians. A similar approach has been adopted by the American Dental Association's Center for Evidence Based Dentistry. The EBD Center offers dental school faculty the opportunity to receive on-site faculty development training in EBP, with courses ranging from 1 to 3 days.

E-Learning is now common both within the predoctoral curriculum and as a means of providing continuing education to practicing dentists. Online course offer advantages in information dissemination without geographic limitations and can scale to large numbers of learners. After participating in an online course, Gruppen and colleagues[54] reported that medical residents, compared with those who did not participate, improved performance in online searching skills, increased the frequency of evidence searches, improved understanding basic biostatistical concepts, and demonstrated greater confidence and enjoyment associated with evidence searching. Similarly, Rohwer and colleagues[56] found that EBM competencies can be adequately presented with online training and showed improvement in knowledge and skills. E-Learners report a "positive attitude" toward online training modules, but they also commonly reported a need for face to face support from tutors. Rohwer and colleagues[57] found E-learning to be effective in improving EBP knowledge and skills, but concluded that combining it with face-to-face learning was needed to improve attitudes and behavior.

Journal clubs are a common approach to teaching scientific literacy in graduate residency programs and among practicing dentists. Both Harris and colleagues[58] and Ahmadi and colleagues[59] assessed among postgraduate (eg, residents) their views of journal clubs compared with more passive learning approaches, such as lectures or printed material. The Ahmandi systematic review found a preference for journal clubs as a process, but neither study found any evidence that they had a sustained impact on patient care.[59] Harris and colleagues[58] found mixed results of the effectiveness of journal clubs, attributing this to poor reporting of the specific methods used to conduct the sessions. Among predoctoral students, journal clubs were reported by Lucia and Swanberg[60] to lead to improved critical thinking and were a preferred learning style among the students. These investigators cautioned that the achievement of the full benefit of journal club participation was dependent on the training and skill of the group facilitator.

Combining various methods seems to offer some advantage in achieving educational goals. Blended or multifaceted interventions provide an opportunity for enhancing the effectiveness of educational interventions. Several systematic reviews have compared multifaceted interventions with single interventions for improving EBP knowledge attitudes and skills. The multifaceted interventions evaluated include various combinations of lectures, computer lab sessions, small group discussions, journal clubs, and assignments. Results show greater improvement with multifaceted intervention sessions.[5,61] The effect size among studies reported in these systematic reviews varied by specific outcomes, with improvement among outcomes of interventions in important areas such as statistical reasoning, critical appraisal skills, self-efficacy, and general attitudes toward research.

Ilic and colleagues[62] found multifaceted interventions to be no more effective than didactic teaching in increasing medical students' competency when assessed using a validated EBM questionnaires. It was, however, significantly more effective at increasing student attitudes toward EBM and self-reported use of EBM in clinical practice. Kyriakoulis and colleagues[61] suggested that, given the various learning styles preferred by students, a multifaceted intervention approach using technology (mobile devices, online simulations) may be well-suited for teaching EBM to early career health students. Coomarasamy and Khan[48] reported that only by integrating EBM teaching with clinical activities was an increase in EBM competency across all domains (knowledge, skills, attitudes and behavior) found in medical postgraduates.

THE PROCESS OF EVIDENCE-BASED PRACTICE

Establishing the understanding that EBP is a clinical activity, teaching the process of EBP is ideally accomplished in the clinic and, as Young and colleagues[5] suggest, needs to be focused on both behavior change (in the student) and clinical outcomes of the patient. Preparing students for evidence-based clinical practice is likely enhanced if it is preceded by clinical case studies as a preclinical exercise. Case studies are generally placed in the context of the dental students' initial exposure to clinical issues through didactic course on diagnosis and treatment planning. Embedding EBP content within a diagnosis and treatment planning course is highly appropriate because this area is the most common in clinical practice where evidence is brought to bear on decision making, thus, reinforcing the clinical relevance of evidence.

PLANNING A CHANGE IN PRACTICE

Lefevre[63] claims that the origins of EBP in the 1990s were based on an unrealistic expectation that physicians would be aware of, read, and scientifically critique all relevant original literature and incorporate the best information into day-to-day practice. This process clearly has not happened and the reasons are the existence of individual and contextual barriers mentioned elsewhere in this article. Studies generally show that the mere dissemination of evidence-based clinical guidelines was ineffective in changing the behavior of health care professionals.[64] Thus, it is important to provide students with a model of how practice behavior can and should change in light of new evidence. Kristensen and colleagues[65] emphasize that teaching EBP requires that the student appreciate the role that individual factors (EBP competency of the clinician) and the context in which the evidence is to be operationalized in daily practice must be understood. The contextual factors include the local culture and leadership that exists in the clinic as well as the attitudes of peers. The overall culture that exists in an clinical setting plays an important role in shaping clinician behavior. In most situations, new evidence will only be implemented by clinicians when it is evaluated in the context of local factors. As a result, these factors can create significant barriers to implementation and must be addressed realistically if the desired behavior change is to be realized.

Assessing the long-term outcomes of various EBP education interventions has not been widely studied. Understandably, in many cases, the time frame for such assessments extends beyond the time students are in training. However, what research that has been done has not shown consistent findings. Ahmadi and colleagues[59] concluded that the EPB skills taught in professional school do not consistently transfer to clinical practice. This is not to say that sustained behavior change never occurs; studies have demonstrated improved clinical practice behavior related to the use of high-quality evidence.[65,66] However, this is not necessarily a predictable outcome of all EBP educational interventions.

The development of implementation science in response to the poor outcomes of standard EBP training has resulted in a rapidly developing knowledge based of what is effective in developing sustainable implementation strategies to ensure that current best evidence is routinely used in patient care. As of yet, there is a lack of what constitutes effective teaching of EBP when the goal is achieving sustained behavior change once students leave the first professional or residency training programs. This area is in need of research on what kind of training actually leads to sustained behavior change.

PRACTICING DENTISTS

Incorporating new evidence into an operating clinical practice can be challenging. Translational research suggests that secondary data sources such as systematic reviews and clinical practice guidelines can be important for translating science into actionable clinical care. However, when these secondary evidence sources challenge existing norms or require substantial changes in clinical care processes or acquiring new clinical skills, formal implementation strategies will need to be used.

Systematic reviews are important as they offer a minimally biased overview of the effectiveness of clinical therapies. Clinical practice guidelines provide clinicians a shortcut to the answer to question about the appropriate application to patient care of evidence derived from systematic reviews. The underlying usefulness of a clinical practice guideline derives from this use as a means of evidence dissemination as well as an adjunct to implementation of best practices. However, guidelines are only useful if they provide objective, unbiased recommendations based on sound science. Training clinicians in assessing the methodologic rigor and appropriateness of a clinical practice guideline to patient care is important, because that process can build trust in the use of guidelines.

When compared with the EBP curriculum in dental schools, any EBP educational program aimed at practicing dentists (those who have completed their formal training programs) will likely need to be adapted in several ways. A first consideration is the difference in knowledge between fully trained dentists and novice students. In the latter case, care must be taken to ensure that language and concepts are appropriate to the novice learner, lest they lose the point of the learning objective when clinical scenarios are used that they cannot yet understand. With the practicing dentists, examples that reflect real-world complexity and important and relevant clinical questions about what is appropriate care should be used to fully engage the learner.

The selection and presentation of material for practicing dentists should be more heavily influenced by adult learning theory. Although the literature on adult learning theory is quite large, several general principles of adult learning theory can be used for EBP developing training.[67]

- Adults need to be involved in the planning and evaluation of their instruction.
- Experience (including mistakes) provides the basis for learning activities. However, it is important to provide an environment where it is safe to make mistakes, without the adult learner being embarrassed or loosing face among colleagues.
- Adults are most interested in learning subjects that have immediate relevance to their job.
- Adult learning is problem centered rather than content oriented.

Studies predicting behavior change in dentists in general are also rare, but some evidence suggests that it must be preceded by attitudinal change.[68] Thus, EBP educational interventions shown to improve attitudes toward EBP would seem to be critical if long-term outcomes to clinical practice are to be realized. There is evidence that training in EBP can improve dentists selection of information sources, favoring higher levels of evidence, and result in changes in patient management.[69–71]

Making EBP training convenient is clearly important, because the time devoted to any training impacts office productivity. Making EBP training understandable for dentists who did not have formal training in statistical and scientific reasoning is also important if they are to take away a clear understanding of how to evaluate and use evidence. Very few EBP educational methods have been evaluated among practicing dentists. Young and colleagues[5] undertook a systematic review of EBP interventions among practicing physicians and found that interactive online courses with guided critical appraisal improved knowledge and appraisal skills. They also found that a short, in-person workshop using problem-based approaches, compared with no intervention, increased knowledge but not appraisal skills.

Our current state of knowledge on what methods are effective for training dentists so that they achieve competency in EBP and routinely search for and implement high-quality evidence in clinical care is essentially nonexistent. This area is in need of urgent research and development. This deficit in understanding dentists' practice behavior and how to impact it is an area that is now being supported by substantial National Institutes of Health research funding. However, we all need to await the results of this research before we can confidently develop interventions for practicing dentists.

SUMMARY

Teaching EBP in dental schools is important because it is an essential component of contemporary dental practice. However, the challenges that exist to implementing an effective EBP educational intervention within a dental school are substantial and require a commitment to the process from both senior leadership as well as across the clinical faculty. The current evidence on teaching effectiveness fails to provide clear guidance on the optimal design of an EBP educational program. Nevertheless, there is a need to move forward with teaching EBP across all levels of dental education (predoctoral, residency, and continuing education). Taking the lessons learned from the existing literature is appropriate and sufficient in many cases to guide educational interventions, particularly those aimed at short-term improvement in knowledge, attitudes, and skills.

Based on current evidence, it is clear that standalone EBP course that are not integrated into the larger clinical curriculum are unlikely to be successful in achieving the desired learning and behavioral outcomes. Combinations of various educational modalities, such as small group discussion, E-learning, case based teaching, computer labs sessions, and journal clubs, when combined with didactic lectures enhance the achievement of educational outcomes. Additional educational research focused on dentistry is needed to understand in which situations various educational approaches offer the best outcomes.

Integrating didactic with clinical teaching seems to be important for improving attitudes, skills, and behaviors. To accomplish effective integration requires a clinical faculty that is well-trained in EBP and routinely models the behavior and holds students accountable for their behavior as it relates to the appropriate use of evidence in managing patients. Training faculty so that they can model the behavior and validly assess students competency implies that resources will need to be expended to create a broad-based and sustainable faculty training program that uses calibrations methods and accommodates faculty turnover.

The importance of achieving EBP competency would be strongly supported by making it required for student graduation. Embedding the knowledge and skills required in clinical examinations and patient management evaluations should also be a part of the evaluation process. Using valid and reliable assessment instruments in this process has been shown to be of value. Hampering the development of optimal EBP educational interventions is the lack of a profession-wide consensus within dentistry as to what constitutes the necessary EBP competencies. Creating such a consensus will improve EPB training by advancing the EBP educational research agenda and improve the development of EBP evaluation instruments.

Studies of the long-term outcomes related to how EBP educational interventions change clinical practice in a sustainable way and how they lead to improved patient outcomes are lacking and additional research is required. As part of this research, the importance of addressing contextual factors for creating and sustaining an effective EBP education program cannot be overstated. If the culture of a dental school does not embrace EBP as valuable in patient care, it is likely that any educational programs will fall short of establishing the desired outcome of creating dentists who are competent in the use of evidence in patient care. Establishing this culture requires strong support from the executive and clinical leadership team and monitoring compliance with EBP teaching goals. Along with this commitment, it must be realized that sufficient resources will need to be committed to establish the infrastructure needed to support the educational program. Such support might include changes to the electronic dental record, the use of periodic reporting of provider performance, and skill development workshops or online training programs for all professional staff.

High-quality health care depends on evidence-informed decision making. Achieving that goal depends on effective EPB educational programs. At present, we stand in great need of more evidence on what constitutes effective teaching for dental students and practicing dentists. Fortunately, there is broad support for developing effective EBP teaching from funding sources and from organized dental education as well as accrediting agencies. These results support the notion that clear guidance on how to conduct effective EBP education is urgently needed.

REFERENCES

1. Institute of Medicine Committee on Quality of Health Care in America. Crossing the quality chasm: a new health system for the 21st century. Washington, DC: National Academy Press; 2001.
2. Guyatt G, Cairns J, Churchill D, et al, Evidence-Based Medicine Working Group. Evidence-based medicine. A new approach to teaching the practice of medicine. JAMA 1992;268(17):2420–5.
3. Dawes M, Summerskill W, Glasziou P, et al. Sicily statement on evidence-based practice. BMC Med Educ 2005;5:1.
4. Cook DJ, Jaeschke R, Guyatt GH. Critical appraisal of therapeutic interventions in the intensive care unit: human monoclonal antibody treatment in sepsis. Journal Club of the Hamilton Regional Critical Care Group. J Intensive Care Med 1992;7: 275–82.
5. Young T, Rohwer A, Volmink J, et al. What are the effects of teaching evidence-based health care (EBHC)? overview of systematic reviews. PLoS One 2014; 9(1):e86706. Available at: https://doi.org/10.1371/journal.pone.0086706.
6. Rosenberg W, Donald A. Evidence based medicine: an approach to clinical problem-solving. BMJ 1995;310:1122–6.
7. Glasziou P, Burls A, Gilbert R. Evidence based medicine and the medical curriculum. BMJ 2008;337:a1253.
8. Hurd PDH. Scientific literacy: new minds for a changing world. Sci Educ 1998;82: 407–16.
9. Shaughnessy AF, Torro JR, Frame KA, et al. Evidence-based medicine and life-long learning competency requirements in new residency teaching standards 10.1136/ebmed-2015-110349. Evid Based Med 2016;21:2.

10. Spallek H, Song M, Polk DE, et al. Barriers to implementing evidence-based clinical guidelines: a survey of early adopters. J Evid Based Dental Pract 2010;10: 195–206.
11. Song M, Spallek H, Polk D, et al. How information systems should support the information needs of general dentists in clinical settings: suggestions from a qualitative study. BMC Med Inform Decis Mak 2010;10:7.
12. Straub-Morarend CL, Wankiiri-Hale CR, Blanchette DR, et al. Evidence-based practice knowledge, perceptions, and behavior: a multiinstitutional, cross-sectional study of a population of U.S. dental students. J Dent Educ 2016;80: 430–8.
13. Bennett S, Tooth L, McKenna K, et al. Perceptions of evidence-based practice: a survey of Australian occupational therapists. Aust Occup Ther J 2003;50:13–22.
14. Fink R, Thompson C, Bonnes D. Overcoming barriers and promoting the use of research in practice. J Nurs Adm 2005;35(3):121–9.
15. Melnyk BM, Fineout-Overholt E, Gallagher-Ford L, et al. The state of evidence-based practice in US nurses: critical implications for nurse leaders and educators. J Nurs Adm 2012;42(9):410–7.
16. Meline T, Paradiso T. Evidence-based practice in schools: evaluating research and reducing barriers. Lang Speech Hear Serv Sch 2003;34:273–83.
17. Glasgow RE, Green LW, Taylor MV, et al. An evidence integration triangle for aligning science with policy and practice. Am J Prev Med 2012;42(6):646–54.
18. Isham A, Bettiol S, Hoang H, et al. A systematic literature review of the information-seeking behavior of dentists in developed countries. J Dent Educ 2016;80(5):569–77.
19. Rangachari P, Rissing P, Rethemeyer K. Awareness of evidence-based practices alone does not translate to implementation: insights from implementation research. Qual Manag Health Care 2013;22(2):117–25.
20. O'Donnell JA, Modesto A, Oakley M, et al. Spallek (2010) Barriers to implementing evidence-based clinical guidelines: a survey of early adopters. J Am Dent Assoc 2014;144:e24–30.
21. Schunk DH. Goal setting and self-efficacy during self-regulated learning. Educ Psychol 2010;25(1):71–86.
22. Schams KA, Kuennen JK. Clinical postconference pedagogy: exploring evidence-based practice with millennial-inspired "building blocks". Creat Nurs 2012;18(1):13–6.
23. Algen B. Pedagogical strategies to teach bachelor students evidence-based practice: a systematic review. Nurse Educ Today 2016;36:255–63.
24. Willingham DT. Critical thinking: why is it so hard to teach? Arts Educ Pol Rev 2008;109:21–32.
25. Reynolds M. Critical thinking and systems thinking: towards a critical literacy for systems thinking in practice. In: Horvath Z, Christopher P, Forte JM, editors. Critical thinking. New York: Nova Science Publishers; 2011. p. 37–68.
26. Zimmerman C. The development of scientific reasoning skills. Developmental Rev 2000;20:99–149.
27. Windish DM, Huot SJ, Green ML. Medicine residents' understanding of the biostatistics and results in the medical literature. JAMA 2007;298:1010–22.
28. Tavris C. Mistakes were made (but not my me). Boston: Houghton Mifflin Harcourt; 2015.
29. Hattie JAC. Visible learning. London: Routledge Taylor & Francis; 2008.
30. Leung K, Trevena L, Waters D. Development of a competency framework for evidence-based practice in nursing. Nurse Educ Today 2016;39:189–96.

31. Sadeghi-Bazargani H, Tabrizi JS, Azami-Aghdash S. Barriers to evidence-based medicine: a systematic review. J Eval Clin Pract 2014;20(6):793–802.

32. Albarqouni L, Hoffman T, Straus S. Core competencies in evidence-based practice for health professionals consensus statement based on a systematic review and Delphi survey. JAMA Netw Open 2018;1(2):e180281.

33. Melnyk BM, Gallagher-Ford L, Long LE, et al. The establishment of evidence-based practice competencies for practicing registered nurses and advanced practice nurses in real-world clinical settings: proficiencies to improve healthcare quality, reliability, patient outcomes, and costs. Worldviews Evid Based Nurs 2014;11:5–15.

34. Marshall TA, Straub-Morarand CL, Buzman-Armstrong S, et al. An approach on defining competency in evidence-based dentistry. Eur J Dent Educ 2018;22: e107–15.

35. CEBM core EBM competencies. Available at: https://webcache.googleusercontent. com/search?q=cache:RLDz-5uKxh0J, https://www.cebm.net/wp-content/uploads/ 2015/09/Core-topics-competencies-for-EBP.docx+&cd=1&hl=en&ct=clnk&gl=us. Accessed August 1, 2018.

36. Galbraith K, Ward A, Heneghan C. A real-world approach to evidence-based medicine in general practice: a competency framework derived from a systematic review and Delphi process. BMC Med Educ 2017;17:78.

37. Ten Cate O, Scheele F. Viewpoint: competency-based postgraduate training: can we bridge the gap between theory and clinical practice? Acad Med 2007;82: 542–7.

38. Shaneyfelt T, Baum KD, Bell D, et al. Instruments for evaluating education in evidence-based practice: a systematic review. JAMA 2006;296(9):1116–27.

39. Fritsche L, Greenhalgh T, Falck-Ytter Y, et al. Do short courses in evidence based medicine improve knowledge and skills? Validation of Berlin questionnaire and before and after study of courses in evidence based medicine. BMJ 2002;325: 1338–2134.

40. Ilic D, Nordin RB, Glasziou P, et al. Development and validation of the ACE tool: assessing medical trainees' competency in evidence based medicine. BMC Med Educ 2014;14:114.

41. Ruzafa-Martinez M, Lopez-Iborra L, Casbas-Moreno T, et al. Development and validation of the competence in evidence based practice questionnaire (EBP-COQ) among nursing students. BMC Med Educ 2013;13:19.

42. Aarons GA, Glisson CH, Hoagwood K, et al. Psychometric properties and U.S. National norms of the Evidence-Based Practice Attitude Scale (EBPAS). Psychol Assess 2010;22(2):356–65.

43. Hisham R, Ng CJ, Liew SM, et al. Development and validation of the Evidence Based Medicine Questionnaire (EBMQ) to assess doctors' knowledge, practice and barriers regarding the implementation of evidence-based medicine in primary care. BMC Fam Pract 2018;19:98. Available at: https://doi.org/10.1186/ s12875-018-0779-5.

44. Hendricson WD, Rugh JD, Hatch JP, et al. Validation of an instrument to assess evidence-based practice knowledge, attitudes, access, and confidence in the dental environment. J Dent Educ 2011;75:131–44.

45. Tilson JK, Kaplan SL, Harris JL, et al. Sicily statement on classification and development of evidence-based practice learning assessment tools. BMC Med Educ 2011;11:78.

46. Ahmadi SF, Baradaran HR, Ahmadi E. Effectiveness of teaching evidence-based medicine to undergraduate medical students: a BEME systematic review. Med Teach 2014;37:21–30.
47. Burn HK, Foley SM. Building a foundation for an evidence-based approach to practice: teaching basic concepts to undergraduate freshman students. J Prof Nurs 2005;21:351–7.
48. Coomarasamy A, Khan KS. What is the evidence that postgraduate teaching in evidence based medicine changes anything? Br Med J 2004;329:1017–9.
49. Khan KS, Coomarasamy A. A hierarchy of effective teaching and learning to acquire competence in evidenced-based medicine. BMC Med Educ 2006;6:59.
50. Profetto-McGrath J. Joanne critical thinking and evidence-based practice. J Prof Nurs 2005;21:364–71.
51. Phillips AC, Lewis LK, McEvoy MP, et al. A systematic review of how studies describe educational interventions for evidence-based practice: stage 1 of the development of a reporting guideline. BMC Med Educ 2014;14:152.
52. Häggman-Laitila A, Mattila LR, Melender AL. Educational interventions on evidence-based nursing in clinical practice: a systematic review with qualitative analysis. Nurse Educ Today 2016;43:50–9.
53. Jonhston JM, Schooling CM, Leung GM. A randomised-controlled trial of two educational modes for undergraduate evidence-based medicine learning in Asia. BMC Med Educ 2009;9:63.
54. Gruppen LD, Rana GK, Arndt TS. A controlled comparison study of the efficacy of training medical students in evidence-based medicine literature searching skills. Acad Med 2005;80:940–4.
55. Ilic D, Maloney S. Methods of teaching medical trainees evidence-based medicine: a systematic review. Med Educ 2014;48:124–35.
56. Rohwer A, Young T, Schalkwyk SV. Effective or just practical? An evaluation of an online postgraduate module on evidence-based medicine (EBM). BMC Med Educ 2013;13:77.
57. Rohwer A, Motaze NV, Rehfuess E, et al. E-learning of evidence-based health care (EBHC) in healthcare professionals: a systematic review. Campbell Systematic Reviews 2017;4. https://doi.org/10.4073/csr.2017.4.
58. Harris J, Kearley K, Heneghan C, et al. Are journal clubs effective in supporting evidence-based decision making? A systematic review. BEME guide No. 16. Med Teach 2011;33:9–23.
59. Ahmadi N, McKenzie ME, MacLean A, et al. Teaching evidence based medicine to surgery residents-is journal club the best format? A systematic review of the literature. J Surg Educ 2012;69:91–100.
60. Lucia VC, Swanberg SM. Utilizing journal club to facilitate critical thinking in pre-clinical medical students. Int J Med Educ 2018;9:7–8.
61. Kyriakoulis K, Patelarou A, Laliotis A, et al. Educational strategies for teaching evidence-based practice to undergraduate health students: systematic review. J Educ Eval Health Prof 2016;13:34.
62. Ilic D, Nordin RB, Glasziou P, et al. A randomised controlled trial of a blended learning education intervention for teaching evidence-based medicine Ilic et al. Ilic et al. BMC Med Educ 2015;15:39.
63. Lefevre M. From authority- to evidence-based medicine: are clinical practice guidelines moving us forward or backward? Ann Fam Med 2017;15(5):4102–212.
64. IOM (Institute of Medicine). Clinical practice guidelines we can trust. Washington, DC: The National Academies Press; 2011.

65. Kristensen N, Nymann C, Konradsen H. Implementing research results in clinical practice- the experiences of healthcare professionals. BMC Health Serv Res 2016;16:48.

66. Straus SE, Green ML, Bell DS, et al. Evaluating the teaching of evidence based medicine: conceptual framework. BMJ 2004;329:1029–32.

67. Knowles M. The adult learner: a neglected species. 3rd edition. Houston (TX): Gulf Publishing; 1984.

68. Yusuf H, Kolliakou A, Ntouva A, et al. Predictors of dentists' behaviours in delivering prevention in primary dental care in England: using the theory of planned behaviour. BMC Health Serv Res 2016;16:44.

69. McGinn T, Seltz M, Korenstein D. A method for real-time, evidence-based general medical attending rounds. Acad Med 2002;77:1150–2.

70. Khan KS, Dwarakanath LS, Pakkal M, et al. Postgraduate journal club as a means of promoting evidence-based obstetrics and gynaecology. J Obstet Gynaecol 1999;19(3):231–4.

71. Haines SJ, Nicholas JS. Teaching evidence-based medicine to surgical subspecialty residents. J Am Coll Surg 2003;197:285–9.

Evidence-Based Dentistry Caries Risk Assessment and Disease Management

Margherita Fontana, DDS, PhD*,
Carlos Gonzalez-Cabezas, DDS, MSD, PhD

KEYWORDS

- Dental caries • Risk assessment • Fluoride • Sealants • Evidence

KEY POINTS

- Dental caries is a multifactorial, dynamic disease process that results from a dysbiosis in the biofilm, driven by exposure to fermentable carbohydrates, which over time can lead to demineralization of dental hard tissues.
- Over time the disease can result in loss of minerals within the tooth structure, or caries lesions, which initially are noncavitated (ie, surface is apparently intact, sometimes referred to as "white spot" lesions), but that eventually might progress to cavitation.
- Modern caries management stresses a conservative and preventive evidence-based philosophy, with personalized disease management, detection and monitoring of caries lesions, and efforts to remineralize and/or arrest lesions whenever possible, that aims to preserve tooth structure and maintain health.

INTRODUCTION

Dental caries is a multifactorial, dynamic disease process that results from a dysbiosis in the biofilm, driven by exposure to fermentable carbohydrates, which over time leads to demineralization of dental hard tissues.[1] In spite of the significant reduction in caries prevalence in many parts of the world, dental caries remains a major public health problem affecting people of all ages.[2] Furthermore, the disease is not equally distributed, with multiple population groups at increased risk.[3,4] If allowed to progress, over time the disease will result in the development of detectable changes in the tooth

Disclosure: Drs M. Fontana and C. Gonzalez-Cabezas do not have any commercial or financial conflicts of interest. They are both active in cariology research. Dr M. Fontana currently receives funding from the National Institutes of Health in areas of caries risk assessment and caries management.
Department of Cariology, Restorative Sciences and Endodontics, University of Michigan School of Dentistry, 1011 North University, Ann Arbor, MI 48109, USA
* Corresponding author. 1011 North University, Room 2393, Ann Arbor, MI 48109.
E-mail address: mfontan@umich.edu

Dent Clin N Am 63 (2019) 119–128
https://doi.org/10.1016/j.cden.2018.08.007
0011-8532/19/© 2018 Elsevier Inc. All rights reserved.

dental.theclinics.com

structure, or caries lesions, which initially are noncavitated (ie, macroscopically intact, sometimes referred to as "white spot" or "incipient" lesions), but that eventually might progress to cavitation.[5,6]

Modern caries management stresses a conservative and preventive evidence-based philosophy, with patient-centered risk-based disease management, early detection of caries lesions, and efforts to remineralize and/or arrest noncavitated lesions that aim to preserve tooth structure and maintain health.[6–8] In support of this philosophy, numerous systems and guidelines have been developed.[9,10] Furthermore, this caries management philosophy is the basis for current cariology education frameworks worldwide.[11,12]

RISK ASSESSMENT

Risk-based prevention and disease management have been recognized as the cornerstones of modern caries management.[13–15] The process of assigning a level of risk of caries involves determining the probability of incidence of caries during a certain time period. It also involves the probability that there will be a change in the severity and/or activity of caries lesions.[14] It is difficult to accurately identify at-risk patients, and the evidence on preventive measures for high-risk individuals is still scarce. In fact, most studies on risk assessment have been conducted in children, and there is very little evidence from adults to help guide how to apply risk assessment models to older populations.[16] However, most experts and organized dentistry organizations contend that when the well-being of the patient is considered, it is more important to carry out a risk assessment incorporating the best available evidence than just doing nothing due to lack of strong evidence.[6] As dental caries is unequally distributed in most populations around the world, including the United States,[3,4] for most dentists it becomes imperative to be able to identify a patient's risk status to be able to develop the most cost-effective and clinically appropriate treatment strategy for that individual.[6] Yet, a survey of clinical practices within a US Practice-Based Research Network suggests that a significant proportion of dentists had yet to adopt treatments based on assessment of caries risk.[17]

Because of the multifactorial nature of the caries process, and the fact that the disease is very dynamic, but not necessarily continuous (eg, lesions can progress and/or regress), risk assessment studies are complex, with a multitude of variables challenging the prediction at different times during life.[15,18,19] Usually, demographic, social, behavioral, and biological variables, along with the clinical/radiographic examination and supplementary tests, are used to develop a caries risk profile or category (eg, low, moderate, or high caries risk). For a clinician, the concepts of assessment of risk and prognosis are important parts of clinical decision-making. In fact, the dentist's overall subjective impression of the patient might have good predictive power for caries risk.[20]

Caries risk tools must be inexpensive and have a high level of accuracy to be cost-effective,[21] and they must be quick and require limited armamentarium to be acceptable.[22] Available caries risk questionnaire tools are, for the most part, expert-opinion based tools, as none have been validated longitudinally in US children, and few in adults.[23] Examples include the caries risk tools of the American Academy of Pediatrics, American Academy of Pediatric Dentistry, American Dental Association (ADA), and the Caries Management by Risk Assessment (CAMBRA).[23–27] Existing data support the conclusion that caries risk can be assessed using only variables easily available from interviewing parents, for example, at periodic medical or dental examinations, without the need of additional clinical testing.[28–30] In addition, "past caries experience" is one of the most powerful predictors of future caries develop-ment.[18,28] However, for monitoring purposes, existing risk tools can be helpful as an objective record of risk included in the patient's chart. A careful analysis including not only past caries experience but also all other risk (eg, presence of plaque, frequent consumption of carbohydrates, decrease in salivary flow rate) and protective factors (eg, exposure to fluorides) will allow the dental team and patient to understand the specific reasons for the caries disease and thus will allow for tailoring a personalized treatment plan and recall interval specifically designed to address the patient's needs.[6,16]

In general, in most risk forms, a low caries risk assessment is based on a combina-tion of the following factors: no caries lesion development or progression for a recent period of time (eg, 3–5 years), low amount of plaque accumulation, low frequency of the patient's sugar intake, no presence of salivary problems, and adequate exposure to protective factors (eg, water fluoridation). In addition, the following factors, whether appearing singly or in combination, would yield a moderate to high risk assessment of caries: the development of new caries lesions, the presence of active lesions, and the placement of restorations due to active disease since the patient's last examination, together with a detrimental change in amount of plaque, incremental frequency of car-bohydrate consumption, decrease in saliva flow, and decrease in exposure to caries protective factors.[6,16]

CARIES MANAGEMENT

Although numerous caries preventive and management therapies are available today, the level of evidence supporting each of the therapies is variable, and clinicians should take that into consideration when developing the management plan. Professional judgment when developing an appropriate caries management plan must take into consideration the patient's risk level, reasons for this increased risk (ie, predisposing risk factors), the patient's readiness for change, and the likelihood of compliance to the different possible therapies. The 2 preventive strategies that remain with the high-est level of supporting evidence are topical fluorides and pit and fissure sealants.[6]

Fluorides

Fluoride has been shown to reduce dental caries incidence consistently in both the pri-mary and permanent dentitions, with the most current evidence strongly suggesting that most of fluoride's effect is topical, by affecting the demineralization-remineralization exchanges between the tooth and the biofilm. Most clinical data for fluoride products and dental caries has focused on the investigation of fluoride's effect on caries lesion prevention. Well-conducted longitudinal clinical studies on use of fluo-ride products to arrest noncavitated or cavitated lesions are much more limited and varied.[6] Systematic reviews have shown that water fluoridation is effective in reducing caries in children and adults,[31] and by 2014, 74.4% of the US population on public wa-ter systems had access to fluoridated water.[32] In some instances in which fluoridated water is not available, prescription of fluoride supplements can be considered for young children. The use of fluoride supplements has been associated with a reduction in caries incidence. The effect is clear in permanent teeth; but the evidence is not as compelling for primary teeth.[33]

Dentifrices with fluoride concentrations of 1000 ppm or above have been shown to reduce dental caries experience,[34,35] with significant in vitro data to additionally show their potential for remineralization of noncavitated lesions, and for some formulations, for example, formulations with fluoride, calcium carbonate, and arginine, additional significant clinical data exist to demonstrate noncavitated lesion arrest.[36] Their use during toothbrushing is probably the most common and effective oral hygiene practice around the world. Due to fluoride's demonstrated efficacy and relative safety, dental and health organizations in the United States and around the world recommend the daily use of fluoridated dentifrices as soon as teeth erupt into the oral cavity. In young children, it is strongly recommended that the use of toothpaste is supervised by an adult. Recommended amounts also tend to be smaller than those used in adults to minimize the risk for development of dental fluorosis.[6,37]

For higher-risk patients, use of additional fluoride products at home (eg, fluoride mouthrinses, high-concentration fluoride dentifrices) or professionally applied (eg, varnishes, gels), can provide additional benefits.[37,38] For example, 5000 ppm fluoride dentifrices (1.1% NaF) are particularly effective in root surface carious lesion prevention and arrest,[39–43] but because there is a dose-response effect of fluoride dentifrices, these high-concentration dentifrices are also commonly considered for patients at higher risk of coronal lesions. Adding a fluoride rinse has been shown to be effective to reduce caries experience in at-risk patients.[38] Professionally applied fluoride products, such as gels and varnishes, are frequently recommended for individuals at higher risk, and are effective for both caries prevention and arrest of noncavitated lesions in primary and permanent teeth.[35] Silver fluoride products (eg, silver diamine fluoride) have also been shown to be effective at arresting cavitated lesions in coronal and root surfaces.[39,44]

Dental Sealants

Sealants are considered one of the most effective evidence-based strategies available to prevent caries lesions on sound occlusal surfaces and to arrest occlusal noncavitated lesions.[45] Yet, although they are recommended and frequently used in school-based public health sealant programs, resulting in median caries reductions of 60%,[46,47] they are unfortunately underutilized in clinical dental settings, even when systematic reviews, including those by the Cochrane Collaboration, support them as either effective or cost-effective to prevent or control caries lesions.[48–51] In fact, the preventive fraction to arrest noncavitated lesions of 71%,[52] is similar to reported values when sealants are used on sound surfaces. And even if clinicians were concerned with sealing in cariogenic bacteria, findings from a systematic review support that bacterial growth is significantly inhibited after sealing bacteria in caries lesions.[53] The most recent evidence-based clinical guidelines for sealant use by the ADA, developed based on a systematic review that focused on studies of sealant materials available in the US market at the time of the review, strongly recommended use of sealants to prevent caries lesions and arrest noncavitated lesions, and conditionally recommended use of sealants over fluoride varnish to prevent caries lesions.[54,55] Regarding which sealant material might be most effective, current systematic reviews by the Cochrane Collaboration and ADA conclude that it is unclear if glass ionomer (GI) sealants are similar to resin-based sealants for caries control.[53] Yet, the ADA expert panel highlighted that it is important to take into account the likelihood of experiencing lack of retention (ie, resin-based materials have significantly higher retention rates over time than GI materials), and the difficulties in being able to obtain a dry field during isolation for sealant placement (ie, GI materials are more hydrophilic), when choosing the type of material to use, and the periodicity of retention checks over time.[54,55]

Sealants have also been used effectively to arrest noncavitated lesions in interproximal surfaces, albeit this procedure is very technique sensitive, and it requires a second visit after tooth separation, as these lesions are normally initially clinically not accessible. As an alternative, infiltration of noncavitated lesions (ie, if not visible by direct observation, assessed based on radiographic depth as radiographically into enamel or outer third of dentin) has been developed as a material and technique to be able to be used in a single dental appointment, and clinical studies and a recent systematic review by the Cochrane Collaboration support that infiltration is a very effective strategy to arrest these lesions in primary and permanent teeth.[56,57]

Sealants have also been found to be effective over time at arresting lesion progression when used on more advanced lesions (ie, microcavitated lesions and/or radiographically extending no more than half-way through the dentin), and repaired yearly.[58] In a recent systematic review and meta-analysis, sealants and minimally invasive restorations led to less-invasive retreatments of more advanced lesions than just preventive care, yet sealants required more repairs over time.[59]

Antimicrobials

Because dental caries results from a dysbiosis in the oral microbiome, restoring balance within that biofilm (through the use of antimicrobials, prebiotics, probiotics, and so forth) has been advocated.[60] Two of the most commonly investigated antimicrobial strategies for caries control and prevention have been chlorhexidine and polyols. Chlorhexidine is a broad-spectrum antimicrobial that has been used in dentistry for a very long time; however, current evidence suggests that chlorhexidine rinses have no beneficial effect in reducing dental caries and should not be routinely recommended.[61] On the other hand, available evidence on chlorhexidine/thymol varnishes applied professionally supports their use for the prevention and management of root caries lesions.[62]

Numerous studies have investigated the anticaries effects of polyols, particularly xylitol, delivered in a wide variety of vehicles, such as chewing gums, lozenges/candies, toothpastes, and wipes. Available evidence shows that xylitol is noncariogenic and has an antimicrobial effect that is dose and frequency dependent. Furthermore, even when the evidence for numerous vehicles is insufficient,[63] systematic reviews have consistently concluded that the regular use of xylitol or polyol-combinations in chewing gum and lozenges can be an effective adjunct in coronal and root caries prevention,[62,64] but whether this is solely because of salivary stimulation or additionally because of the antimicrobial effects of the polyol, or whether it is substituting what otherwise would have been sugar ingestion, is less clear.

Probiotics have been used in dentistry for caries control in both children and adults. Most of the published studies have used probiotics strains originally targeted to the gastrointestinal tract. Although the evidence is still limited and inconsistent, and most of the tested products are experimental and not available for commercial use yet, this may be a promising future approach to modulate biofilm dysbiosis.[65]

Calcium-Based Strategies

Even though there has been a reduction in caries experience in many places around the world in the past many decades, dental caries is still a significant public health problem affecting people of all ages,[66] and even with regular fluoride use, carious lesions can still develop if risk factors are present. These challenges, among others, have supported the need for continued research into cost-effective strategies for caries prevention and management that could work as a booster/supplement or as an alternative to fluoride. A variety of products containing calcium in different forms (eg, calcium attached to casein derivatives, calcium sodium phosphosilicate) have been introduced to aid with remineralization. The evidence supporting the clinical efficacy of these products is still either limited or inconsistent.[67] Recent systematic reviews have concluded that although there are clinical studies supporting the remineralization potential of some of these formulations (eg, casein phosphopeptide amorphous calcium phosphate) over a placebo, there is yet insufficient evidence from clinical trials demonstrating that any of these products prevent dental caries or arrest caries lesions better than fluoride, or that they consistently enhance fluoride's efficacy for caries prevention and arrest noncavitated lesions.[68] In fact, some longitudinal clinical studies have concluded that 10% casein phosphopeptide and amorphous calcium phosphate paste is not effective to arrest or remineralize noncavitated caries lesions.[69,70] On the other hand, the use of a prebiotic, such as arginine, to modulate dysbiotic dental biofilms by increasing plaque pH, in combination with fluoride, has consistently shown an ability to enhance the anticaries and remineralization effects of fluoride in 8 clinical trials.[36] Yet, even when the evidence is promising and consistently supportive, all the trials have been conducted by the manufacturers, and most are short term, thus there is a need for longer-term trials, also by other groups.[68]

Management of Cavitated Lesions

Cavitated caries lesions that limit regular dental plaque removal are likely to progress and generally require restorative treatment as part of the caries management for that patient.[71] However, as stated previously, silver fluoride products (eg, silver diamine fluoride) have also been shown to be effective at arresting cavitated lesions in coronal and root surfaces.[39,44]

The main objective of restoring cavitated lesions, from a disease management perspective, is to stop the caries activity of the lesion and the restoration of a cleansable and functional tooth surface. The introduction of adhesive materials with mechanical and physical properties has revolutionized the design of cavity preparations allowing for much more conservative restorative dentistry.[6] Cavitated caries lesions should be restored using minimally invasive principles minimizing the removal of tissue, with the goal of preserving as much tooth structure as possible.

An International Caries Consensus Collaboration presented recommendations on terminology and on carious tissue removal and managing cavitated carious lesions.[72] They recommended the level of hardness (soft, leathery, firm, and hard dentine) as the criterion for determining the clinical consequences of the disease and defined new strategies to carious tissue removal: (1) selective removal of carious tissue, including selective removal to soft dentine and selective removal to firm dentine; (2) stepwise removal, including initially selective removal to soft dentine, and at a second appointment 6 to 12 months later selective removal to firm dentine; and (3) nonselective removal to hard dentine, formerly known as complete caries removal (technique no longer recommended). Furthermore, they suggested controlling the disease in cavitated carious lesions should be attempted using methods that are aimed at biofilm removal or control first. Only when cavitated carious lesions either are noncleansable or can no longer be sealed are restorative interventions indicated. Carious tissue should be removed purely to create conditions for long-lasting restorations. Bacterially contaminated or demineralized tissues close to the pulp do not need to be removed. The evidence and, therefore, these recommendations support less-invasive carious lesion management, delaying entry to, and slowing down, the restorative cycle by preserving tooth tissue and retaining teeth long-term.[72]

SUMMARY

Patient-centered "personalized" prevention and management of dental caries should be based on restoring the balance in the oral environment, with the goal of preserving tooth structure, using best evidence available and taking into consideration the dentist's expertise and individual needs of the patient.[6] Although there is significant evidence supporting many of the individual components of this caries management philosophy, such as use of fluorides and sealants for caries prevention and management,[7,9] there is scarcity of data in the literature to demonstrate the cost-effectiveness of this system approach when used in general dental practice, especially among adult patients. Yet, available data suggest that a risk-based caries management system, in which risk is based on disease experience, and management uses evidence-based approaches, such as use of sealants and fluoride varnishes (with frequency tailored on risk), can be effective at decreasing restorative needs over time in adult populations in private practice settings.[8,73]

REFERENCES

1. Fontana M, Wolff M, Featherstone JBD. Introduction to ICNARA 3. Adv Dent Res 2018;29(1):3.
2. Kassebaum NJ, Bernabe E, Dahiya M, et al. Global burden of untreated caries: a systematic review and meta regression. J Dent Res 2015;1–9.
3. Dye BA, Thornton-Evans G, Li X, et al. Dental caries and sealant prevalence in children and adolescents in the United States, 2011-2012. NCHS Data Brief 2015;191:1–8.
4. Dye BA, Tan S, Smith V, et al. Trends in oral health status: United States, 1988-1994 and 1999-2004. Vital Health Stat 11 2007;(248):1–92.
5. Fontana M, Young D, Wolff M, et al. Defining dental caries for 2010 and beyond. Dent Clin North Am 2010;54:423–40.
6. Fontana M, Gonzalez-Cabezas C, Fitzgerald M. Cariology for the 21st century—current caries management concepts for dental practice. J Mich Dent Assoc 2013;April:32–40.
7. Slayton RL, Fontana M, Young D, et al. Dental caries management in children and adults. In: discussion paper. Washington, DC: National Academy of Medicine; 2016. Available at: https://nam.edu/wp-content/uploads/2016/09/Dental-Caries-Management-in-Children-and-Adults.pdf. Accessed May 6, 2018.
8. Fontana M, González-Cabezas C. Noninvasive caries risk-based management in private practice settings may lead to reduced caries experience over time. J Evid Based Dent Pract 2016;16(4):239–42.
9. Ismail AI, Tellez M, Pitts NB, et al. Caries management pathways preserve dental tissues and promote oral health. Community Dent Oral Epidemiol 2013;41(1):e12–40.
10. Pitts NB, Ekstrand KR, ICDAS Foundation. International Caries Detection and Assessment System (ICDAS) and its International Caries Classification and Management System (ICCMS)—methods for staging of the caries process and enabling dentists to manage caries. Community Dent Oral Epidemiol 2013;41(1):41–52.
11. Fontana M, Guzman-Armnstrong S, Schenkel AB, et al. Development of a core curriculum in cariology for US dental schools. J Dent Educ 2016;80(6):705–20.
12. Schulte AG, Pitts NB, Huysmans MC, et al. European Core Curriculum in Cariology for undergraduate dental students. Eur J Dent Educ 2011;15(1):9–17.
13. Featherstone JDB. The caries balance: contributing factors and early detection. J Calif Dent Assoc 2003;31(2):129–33.
14. Fontana M, Zero D. Assessing patients' caries risk. J Am Dent Assoc 2006;137(9):1231–40.
15. Fontana M. The clinical, environmental and behavioral factors that foster early childhood caries. Ped Dent 2015;37:217–25.

16. Fontana M, Gonzalez-Cabezas C. Minimal intervention dentistry part 2. Caries risk assessment in adults. Br Dent J 2012;213:447–51.
17. Riley JL III, Gordan VV, Rindal DB, et al. Preferences for caries prevention agents in adult patients: findings from the dental practice–based research network. Community Dent Oral Epidemiol 2010;38:360–70.
18. Mejàre I, Axelsson S, Dahlén G, et al. Caries risk assessment. A systematic review. Acta Odontol Scand 2014;72(2):81–91.
19. Twetman S, Fontana M. Patient caries risk assessment. Monogr Oral Sci 2009;21: 91–101.
20. Disney JA, Graves RC, Stamm JW, et al. The University of North Carolina caries risk assessment study: further developments in caries risk prediction. Community Dent Oral Epidemiol 1992;20:64–75.
21. Quinonez RB, Crall J. Caries risk assessment. In: Berg J, Slayton R, editors. Early childhood oral health. IA: Wiley-Blackwell; 2009. p. 170–97.
22. Stamm J, Disney J, Graves R, et al. The University of North Carolina caries risk assessment study. I: rationale and content. J Public Health Dent 1988;48:225–32.
23. Featherstone JDB, Chaffee BW. The evidence for caries management by risk assessment (CAMBRA®). Adv Dent Res 2018;29(1):9–14.
24. American Academy of Pediatric Dentistry. Guideline on caries-risk assessment and management for infants, children, and adolescents. Reference Manual 2014;37(6):15–6.
25. American Dental Association. Caries form (Patients >6). 2008. Available at: http://www.ada.org/~/media/ADA/Science%20and%20Research/Files/topic_caries_over6. ashx. Accessed May 6, 2018.
26. American Dental Association. Caries form (Patients 0-6). 2008. Available at: https://www.ada.org/~/media/ADA/Member%20Center/FIles/topics_caries_under6.ashx. Accessed May 6, 2018.
27. American Academy of Pediatrics. Oral health risk assessment tool. Available at: https://www.aap.org/en-us/Documents/oralhealth_RiskAssessmentTool.pdf. Accessed May 6, 2018.
28. Zero D, Fontana M, Lennon AM. Clinical applications and outcomes of using indicators of risk in caries management. J Dent Educ 2001;65(10):1126–32.
29. Fontana M, Jackson R, Eckert G, et al. Identification of caries risk factors in toddlers. J Dent Res 2011;90(2):209–14.
30. Fontana M, Santiago E, Eckert GJ, et al. Risk factors of caries progression in a Hispanic school-age population. J Dent Res 2011;90:1189–96.
31. Iheozor-Ejiofor Z, Worthington HV, Walsh T, et al. Water fluoridation for the prevention of dental caries. Cochrane Database Syst Rev 2015;(6):CD010856.
32. Centers for Disease Control and Prevention. Water fluoridation data & statistics. Available at: https://www.cdc.gov/fluoridation/statistics/index.htm. Accessed May 6, 2018.
33. Tubert-Jeannin S, Auclair C, Amsallem E, et al. Fluoride supplements (tablets, drops, lozenges or chewing gums) for preventing dental caries in children. Cochrane Database Syst Rev 2011;(12):CD007592.
34. Walsh T, Worthington HV, Glenny AM, et al. Fluoride toothpastes of different concentrations for preventing dental caries in children and adolescents. Cochrane Database Syst Rev 2010;(1):CD007868.
35. Marinho VC, Worthington HV, Walsh T, et al. Fluoride varnishes for preventing dental caries in children and adolescents. Cochrane Database Syst Rev 2013;(7):CD002279.

36. Wolff MS, Schenkel AB. The anticaries efficacy of a 1.5% arginine and fluoride toothpaste. Adv Dent Res 2018;29(1):93–7.
37. Weyant RJ, Tracy SL, Anselmo TT, et al. Topical fluoride for caries prevention: executive summary of the updated clinical recommendations and supporting systematic review. J Am Dent Assoc 2013;144(11):1279–91.
38. Marinho VC, Chong LY, Worthington HV, et al. Fluoride mouthrinses for preventing dental caries in children and adolescents. Cochrane Database Syst Rev 2016;(7):CD002284.
39. Wierichs RJ, Meyer-Lueckel H. Systematic review on noninvasive treatment of root caries lesions. J Dent Res 2015;94(2):261–71.
40. Lynch E, Baysan A, Ellwood R, et al. Effectiveness of two fluoride dentifrices to arrest root carious lesions. Am J Dent 2000;13(4):218–20.
41. Baysan A, Lynch E, Ellwood R, et al. Reversal of primary root caries using dentifrices containing 5,000 and 1,100 ppm fluoride. Caries Res 2001;35(1):41–6.
42. Ekstrand K, Martignon S, Holm-Pedersen P. Development and evaluation of two root caries controlling programmes for home-based frail people older than 75 years. Gerodontology 2008;25(2):67–75.
43. Ekstrand KR, Poulsen JE, Hede B, et al. A randomized clinical trial of the anticaries efficacy of 5,000 compared to 1,450 ppm fluoridated toothpaste on root caries lesions in elderly disabled nursing home residents. Caries Res 2013; 47(5):391–8.
44. Gao SS, Zhang S, Mei ML, et al. Caries remineralisation and arresting effect in children by professionally applied fluoride treatment—a systematic review. BMC Oral Health 2016;16:12.
45. Fontana M. Caries sealing in permanent teeth. In: Schwendicke F, editor. Management of deep carious lesions. Springer International Publishing; 2018. p. 93–112 [Chapter: 7].
46. Truman BI, Gooch BF, Sulemana I, et al. Task Force on Community Preventive Services: reviews of evidence on interventions to prevent dental caries, oral and pharyngeal cancers, and sports-related craniofacial injuries. Am J Prev Med 2002;23:21–54.
47. Gooch BF, Griffin SO, Gray SK, et al. Preventing dental caries through school-based sealant programs: updated recommendations and reviews of evidence. J Am Dent Assoc 2009;140(11):1356–65.
48. Griffin S, Naavaal S, Scherrer C, et al. School-based dental sealant programs prevent cavities and are cost-effective. Health Aff (Millwood) 2016;35(12): 2233–40.
49. Ahovuo-Saloranta A, Hiiri A, Nordblad A, et al. Pit and fissure sealants for preventing dental decay in the permanent teeth of children and adolescents. Cochrane Database Syst Rev 2008;(4):CD001830.
50. Bravo M, Montero J, Bravo JJ, et al. Sealant and fluoride varnish in caries: a randomized trial. J Dent Res 2005;84(12):1138–43.
51. Ahovuo-Saloranta A, Forss H, Walsh T, et al. Sealants for preventing dental decay in the permanent teeth. Cochrane Database Syst Rev 2013;(3):CD001830.
52. Griffin SO, Oong E, Kohn W, Vidakovic B, Gooch BF, CDC Dental Sealant Systematic Review Work Group, Bader J, Clarkson J, Fontana MR, Meyer DM, Rozier RG, Weintraub JA, Zero DT. The effectiveness of sealants in managing caries lesions. J Dent Res 2008;87:169–74.
53. Oong EM, Griffin SO, Kohn WG, et al. The effect of dental sealants on bacteria levels in caries lesions. A review of the evidence. J Am Dent Assoc 2008;139: 271–8.

54. Wright JT, Tampi MP, Graham L, et al. Evidence-based clinical practice guidelines for the use of pit-and-fissure sealants: a report of the American Dental Association and the American Academy of Pediatric Dentistry. J Am Dent Assoc 2016;147(8):672–82.
55. Wright JT, Tampi MP, Graham L, et al. Sealants for preventing and arresting pit-and-fissure occlusal caries in primary and permanent molars: a systematic review of randomized controlled trials—A report from the American Dental Association and the American Academy of Pediatric Dentistry. J Am Dent Assoc 2016; 147(8):631–45.
56. Meyer-Luckel H, Balbach A, Schikowsky C, et al. Pragmatic RCT on efficacy of proximal resin infiltration. J Dent Res 2016;95(5):531–6.
57. Dorri M, Sunne SM, Walsh T, et al. Micro-invasive interventions for managing proximal dental decay in primary and permanent teeth. Cochrane Database Syst Rev 2015;(11):CD010431.
58. Fontana M, Platt JA, Eckert GJ, et al. Monitoring of caries lesion severity under sealants for 44 months. J Dent Res 2014;93:1070–5.
59. Schwendicke F, Jäger AM, Paris S, et al. Treating pit-and-fissure caries: a systematic review and network meta-analysis. J Dent Res 2015;94(4):522–33.
60. Marsh PD. In sickness and in health—what does the oral microbiome mean to us? An ecological perspective. Adv Dent Res 2018;29(1):60–5.
61. Walsh T, Oliveira-Neto JM, Moore D. Chlorhexidine treatment for the prevention of dental caries in children and adolescents. Cochrane Database Syst Rev 2015;(4):CD008457.
62. Rethman MP, Beltran-Aguilar ED, Billings RJ, et al, American Dental Association Council on Scientific Affairs Expert Panel on Nonfluoride Caries-Preventive Agents. Nonfluoride caries-preventive agents: executive summary of evidence-based clinical recommendations. J Am Dent Assoc 2011;142(9):1065–71.
63. Riley P, Moore D, Ahmed F, et al. Xylitol-containing products for preventing dental caries in children and adults. Cochrane Database Syst Rev 2015;(3):CD010743.
64. Fontana M, Gonzalez-Cabezas C. Are we ready for definitive clinical guidelines on xylitol/polyol use? Adv Dent Res 2012;24(2):123–8.
65. Gruner D, Paris S, Schwendicke F. Probiotics for managing caries and periodontitis: systematic review and meta-analysis. J Dent 2016;48:16–25.
66. Broadbent JM, Foster Page LA, Thomson WM, et al. Permanent dentition caries through the first half of life. Br Dent J 2013;215(7):E12.
67. Fontana M. Enhancing fluoride: clinical human studies of alternatives or boosters for caries management. Caries Res 2016;50(Suppl 1):22–37.
68. Gonzalez-Cabezas C, Fernandez CE. Recent advances in remineralization therapies for caries lesions. Adv Dent Res 2018;29(1):55–9.
69. Altenburger MJ, Gmeiner B, Hellwig E, et al. The evaluation of fluorescence changes after application of casein phosphopeptides (CPP) and amorphous calcium phosphate (ACP) on early carious lesions. Am J Dent 2010;23(4):188–92.
70. Sitthisettapong T, Phantumvanit P, Huebner C, et al. Effect of CPP-ACP paste on dental caries in primary teeth: a randomized trial. J Dent Res 2012;91(9):847–52.
71. Kidd AM. Clinical threshold for carious tissue removal. Dent Clin North Am 2010; 54:541–9.
72. Schewendicke F, Frenchen J, Bjørndal L, et al. Managing carious lesions: recommendations on carious tissue removal. Adv Dent Res 2016;28:58–67.
73. Evans RW, Clark P, Jia N. The caries management system: are preventive effects sustained postclinical trial? Community Dent Oral Epidemiol 2016;44(2):188–97.

Translational Research
Bringing Science to the Provider Through Guideline Implementation

Julie Frantsve-Hawley, PhD[a],*, D. Brad Rindal, DDS[b]

KEYWORDS

- Dissemination • Implementation • Dissemination and implementation
- Knowledge translation • Translational research • Implementation science
- Evidence-based dentistry • Evidence-based medicine

KEY POINTS

- The Institutes of Medicine has documented quality gaps in medical care, including variation in practice patterns. Similar quality gaps and practice variation exist in dentistry.
- Evidence-based health care was developed to address quality and practice variation, including evidence summary tools and dissemination tactics, such as evidence-based guidelines.
- Because dissemination of evidence is not generally sufficient to instill change in clinical practice, the field of implementation science was developed to facilitate research regarding barriers and facilitators of provider behavior change and to develop and evaluate intervention strategies that lead to improved, evidence-based care.

THE IMPORTANCE OF TRANSLATING EVIDENCE INTO PRACTICE

In 2001, the National Academies of Science's Institute of Medicine (IOM)[1] issued a report ("Crossing the Quality Chasm") documenting some of the quality of care shortcomings of the US health care system and proposing reforms for the twenty-first century. The IOM identified significant gaps in the quality of care delivered throughout the United States, and characterized the gaps as *overuse*, *underuse*, and *misuse*. For example, an assessment of 3000 medical practices or treatments found that slightly more than a third were effective or likely to be effective, 15% to 25% were unneeded or potentially harmful,[2–4] and 50% were of unknown effectiveness.[4]

Overuse refers to the continued use of treatments that are known to be ineffective, or where the known harms exceed the known benefits.[5] Systematic reviews on

Disclosure Statement: The authors have nothing to disclose.
[a] Department of Guidelines & Publishing, American College of Chest Physicians, 2595 Patriot Boulevard, Glenview, IL 60026, USA; [b] HealthPartners Institute, 3311 East Old Shakopee Road, Bloomington, MN 55425, USA
* Corresponding author.
E-mail address: frantsvehawley@gmail.com

Dent Clin N Am 63 (2019) 129–144
https://doi.org/10.1016/j.cden.2018.08.008
0011-8532/19/© 2018 Elsevier Inc. All rights reserved.

overuse identified several areas of consistent overuse in medicine, including the use of transesophageal echocardiography in patients with stroke, trends of increased use of computed tomography scans in the emergency department, and overuse of antidepressants in children.[6,7] The proliferation of treatments in which harms exceed benefit include treatment for early-stage prostate cancer, oxygen for patients with moderate chronic obstructive pulmonary disease, nutritional interventions for inpatients with malnutrition, and antibiotic overuse.[7] Overuse of screening and diagnostic testing is known to cause false-positive results and overdiagnosis, and overtreatment, with both medical therapies and procedural interventions, and places patients at risk of unnecessary adverse events.[6–8] A common example of overuse in dentistry is the practice of prescribing prophylactic antibiotics for patients with prosthetic joints who are undergoing dental procedure. Recent guidelines based on the current best evidence recommend against this practice based on lack of association between dental procedures and prosthetic joint infection, and increased risk of harms, including antibiotic resistance, adverse drug reactions, and costs, associated with antibiotic use.[9]

Underuse refers to the failure to provide treatments known to be effective and medically necessary. For example, in the United States there is an underuse of screening for serious diseases such as breast, colon, and lung cancer, with rates varying substantially by racial/ethnic, economic, and geographic status.[10,11] These disparities in who receives screening leads to important disparities in health outcomes. When patients fail to consistently receive known effective care, patient and population health outcomes suffer. An important example of underuse in dentistry is the low rates of pit-and-fissure sealant use with patients at high risk of developing occlusal caries or with early noncavitated lesions that can be successfully managed with the need for operative intervention. This underuse occurs despite robust evidence of their effectiveness in primary and secondary caries prevention.[12,13]

Misuse occurs when care is not provided correctly and safely and can be described as medical errors. One important example of misuse occurs when medications are prescribed for the wrong purpose, or not consistent with prescribing recommendations (dose and duration), leading to unnecessary adverse events.[14–17] The current opioid epidemic in the United States is a prominent example of the harms incurred with the misuse of drugs resulting in large personal and societal costs.[17–19]

Collectively, overuse, underuse, and misuse represent examples of what is termed the *Know-Do Gap*. The Know-Do Gap is simply the difference between what we know (the evidence) and what we do (current practice patterns). In an ideal situation, practice patterns should be consistent with evidence (Knowing = Doing), but unfortunately this is not consistently the case and leads to the Know-Do Gap.

What factors contribute to the development of a Know-Do Gap? Research suggests that the timeline from the creation of relevant evidence until it is adopted into routine practice can be surprisingly long. For example, one study estimated it took an average of 17 years for high-quality evidence to enter routine clinical practice.[20,21] This may be due, in part, to the current model used for evidence transfer or dissemination. At many points, inefficiencies occur in the dissemination and adoption of information, contributing importantly to a failure of clinicians to willingly embrace new ideas. Glasziou and Haynes[22] identified 7 stages at which the translation of evidence into routine clinical practice can break down, and failure at any of the following translational stages will impede the adoption into practice of new evidence (**Fig. 1**): *awareness* of the evidence, *acceptance* of the evidence, determination if the evidence is *applicable* to the patient/population; *ability* to carry out the intervention; *act* on the evidence in use it in the decision-making process; *agreed* to by the patient, and patient/provider *adherence*. New knowledge is never completely translated through any of these steps. For

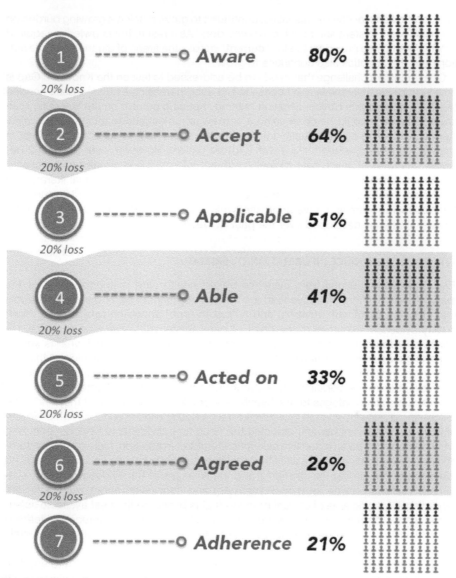

Fig. 1. Pathway from research to practice. At each step, approximately 20% of scientific evidence "leaks" and fails to proceed to the next step. This results in only 21% of scientific evidence being incorporated into patient care. (*Adapted from* Glasziou P, Haynes B. The paths from research to improved health outcomes. ACP J Club 2005;142(2):A8–10; with permission.)

example, if one imagines that 20% of the information at each step fails to transfer, the result will be that only approximately 21% of the knowledge generated would effectively be translated and ultimately adopted into routine clinical practice.

Adding to the Know-Do Gap is the rapid advancements ongoing in medical and dental science, which so often are accompanied by increasing complexity in the process of care delivery. Additionally, the number of individuals requiring such complex care, particularly for chronic diseases, continues to grow, placing a growing burden on the health care system and health care providers. As a result, the knowledge required among health care providers to stay "current" across the areas of diagnostics, prevention, and therapeutics also continues to grow.

One important challenge that needs to be addressed to lessen the Know-Do Gap is how to improve awareness and access to the ever-increasing evidence-base needed to inform appropriate clinical decision making. Keeping current on the scientific literature historically could be done using a somewhat unfocused reading of the clinical literature, drawing on high-quality information sources, "just in case" some kernel of wisdom could be gleaned for use with a future patient. However, over the past 2 decades, the rates at which new clinically relevant information is created and disseminated has reached a point where effectively reading the primary clinical literature in almost any health care field would be infeasible for most busy clinicians.[23] Fortunately, translational researchers have addressed this issue of "information overload" using several strategies developed over the past 20 years.

STRATEGIES TO REDUCE INFORMATION OVERLOAD

Two major contributions from evidence-based health care methodologists for the management of information overload are the development of secondary data analysis methods (eg, systematic reviews) and a "just-in-time" approach to accessing high-quality evidence resources at the point of care. Systematic reviews summarize evidence on important topics and allow clinicians to rapidly understand what is known regarding a specific area of clinical care. Systematic reviews are developed through a rigorous and transparent scientific methodology to identify, appraise, and synthesize all relevant literature pertaining to a particular clinical question. Systematic reviews provide several advantages for the health care provider. The first is that they endeavor to identify all relevant scientific evidence on a particular clinical question, which in and of itself is a significant benefit, reducing the need for individuals to seek out and read what at times can be an extensive scientific literature. In addition, high-quality systematic reviews critically appraise all of the included studies, providing an assessment and transparency regarding the strengths and weaknesses of the evidence. Finally, systematic reviews provide an overall summary and conclusion about what is known regarding a specific area of clinical practice that is based on the best available scientific evidence. Systematic reviews thus provide a highly efficient approach to reading the clinical literature, while providing evidence that is minimally biased and thus likely validly describes the true benefits and harms of clinical interventions.

The other major advancement supporting an evidence-based approach to practice is the "just-in-time" attitude to information seeking. In this approach, clinicians with training in evidence-based practice address clinical questions that arise during routine patient care by using their ability to efficiently seek out high-quality evidence as an adjunct to clinical decision making. This was the original approach developed by Sackett[24] and Guyatt at McMaster University in the 1990s,[25,26] made possible by the development of online evidence databases (eg, PubMed) and associated search engines. Both of these concepts, evidence summarization via systematic reviews and rapid retrieval of relevant and high-quality evidence, when needed to inform clinical decisions, have the potential to contribute substantially to the quality of care delivered. However, the underlying concept of evidence-based practice that these ideas support are ad hoc in nature and depend on a willing and well-trained clinician to retrieve appropriate evidence. More recently, efforts to systematize the transfer of scientific information into clinical practice has been developing, with the aim of ensuring

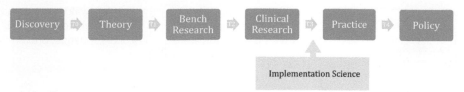

Fig. 2. Domains of translational research.

that all clinicians understand the current best evidence and appropriately apply it to all patients when indicated. This is the domain of translational research and represents a shift in focus from ad hoc, individual provider–driven application of clinical evidence to a system-level approach. The goal of scaling up the application of appropriate evidence to a system level and making it a routine part of clinical practice across an entire health care system has as its aim improvement in both patient and population health as well as increased efficiency in the delivery of care.

FIVE STAGES OF TRANSLATIONAL RESEARCH

In general terms, translational research refers to the study of ways of applying scientific research that lead to improved human health and well-being. This involves the entire process of transferring basic science information into knowledge that can be used clinically and is often referred to as the process of moving scientific discovery from "bench to bedside." Translational research can be thought of as occurring in 5 stages, known as Translational Research Stages 0 to 4, or abbreviated as T0, T1, T2, T3, and T4 (**Fig. 2**).[27,28]

Along this continuum, T3 research focuses on the translation of evidence into routine clinical practice and is thus the domain of most relevance to evidence-based medicine (and dentistry). T3 research endeavors to improve the uptake of evidence into routine practice, through, among other things, the study of evidence dissemination and implementation. Clinical practice guidelines provide a good example of fruits of this area of study, and along with other similar tools aimed at synthesizing evidence, it has become clear that the process leading to adaptation of guidelines by practitioners and health care systems warrants study as its own area of research. This has led over the past 20 years to the birth of a new domain of research.

CLINICAL PRACTICE GUIDELINES

One of the most important strategies developed to translate current scientific evidence into routine clinical practice has been the development of clinical practice guidelines (CPGs). CPGs are defined as "systematically developed statements to assist practitioner and patient decisions about appropriate health care for specific clinical circumstances."[29] Guidelines are developed through a standardized and rigorous process (**Fig. 3**), and leverage evidence available through systematic reviews to develop practical recommendations of how the science can be considered for usage in a practice setting. When implemented, guidelines can reduce inappropriate practice variation, promote use of effective interventions, reduce use of ineffective therapies, and improve patient and population health outcomes.[30] Ultimately, they are a significant resource that helps to ensure that patients receive evidence-based care.

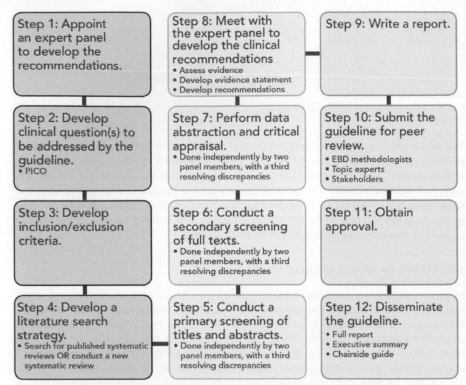

Fig. 3. Guideline development process. EBD, evidence-based dentistry; PICO, P = patient, problem, or population, I = intervention, C = comparison, control, or comparator, O = outcome. (*From* Frantsve-Hawley J. Evidence-based dentistry for the dental hygienist. 1st edition. Hanover Park (IL): Quintessence Publishing; 2014. p. 131; with permission.)

Nonetheless, publishing a clinical guideline does not ensure a change in clinical practice,[31] and indeed, a review of 59 published evaluations of clinical guidelines concluded that guidelines could improve clinical practice, but the size of the improvements in performance varied considerably.[32] Although guidelines can provide a reliable resource for providers in an attempt to bridge the quality chasm, they are not routinely adopted.[33–35] Reasons for this include the following: overlapping and redundant guidelines developed by different organizations, the currency of guidelines that may quickly become outdated as new evidence arises, lack of awareness, complexity, and lack of personal or system-level ability to implement the guideline.[33,36,37] The use of specific strategies overcomes barriers to adoption, and to implement research-based recommendations appears necessary to change practice, as more-intensive efforts are generally more successful.[38]

Barriers to adopting CPG recommendations specific to dentistry include the changing current practice model, colleagues' actions, trust in the validity or currency of the evidence, lack of clarity or contradictory information across various information sources, and personal experience that is perceived to contradict the recommendations.[39,40] Financial barriers (eg, insurance reimbursement) are also created.

Importantly, social environment is a factor impacting behavior, and these results suggest that the peer influence was strongly associated with changing provider behavior, as was the perception of what was the prevailing standard of practice.[41]

Together, this information on barriers to adopting evidence-based recommendations provides insight into why proving information alone is often not sufficient to instill changes in practice patterns. Targeted and strategic efforts are required to translate science into practice.

IMPLEMENTATION SCIENCE

As described in **Fig. 2**, implementation science fits within the T3 phase of translational research. Implementation science comprises both dissemination and implementation. The terms *dissemination* and *implementation* are defined in **Table 1**.[42–44] As opposed to diffusion of knowledge, which occurs passively, dissemination uses specific tactics to increase awareness about scientific evidence. Implementation takes this to the next step by developing and evaluating specific strategies aimed at changing provider behavior in concordance with the evidence to the point at which the evidence-based treatment becomes routine and sustainable. Taken together, implementation science is targeted toward an increasing awareness and utilization of evidence to improve practice through individual, organizational, and policy-level change.[45–47] The ultimate goal of implementation science is to develop permanent, sustained improvements in practice patterns through removing barriers to adoption and ultimately changing the culture around care delivery.[48,49]

Seeking a change in practice pattern is dependent on a change in provider behavior. Before attempting to change practice patterns, it is important to first assess the clinical and administrative environments regarding the perceived need for change (ie, how large is the Know-Do Gap) and the understanding of professional staff as to the existence of such a gap. This relates to the willingness of professional staff to engage in change. This initial assessment will provide important guidance for selecting subsequent implementation strategies and can then be followed up by identification of specific structural barriers that prevent the desired behavior change as well as facilitators that can promote that change. The barriers to organizational change are extensive. Most "systems" (ie, organizations) are stable and self-sustaining. Thus, change requires interventions that address the factors that control that stability. Failure to address the barriers will usually result in partial or complete failure to implement desired change. Each organization or system is, to a large part, unique, and so will be the barriers to change. Implementation science, however, provides insight in to broad categories that must be considered when looking at system-level implementations. These categories include financial disincentives, time constraints, patient expectations, social norms, perceived standard of practice, potential for liability or tort claims, influence of key opinion leaders, professional staff knowledge and skill, and attitudes around confidence in ability to change.[50] Facilitators are typically complementary to barriers, and include an environment in which providers have the confidence and ability to change behavior, financial incentives are provided, information is accessible and understandable, and the health care system provides the time and resources needed to illicit the desired practice change. These barriers and facilitators can occur at multiple levels, including at the provider level, clinic level, and at the health care system level.[50–53]

As the premier funder of new knowledge around health and disease, the National Institutes of Health has great interest in ensuring that the products (ie, new knowledge) of their investments are effectively translated into improvements in clinical practice and patient health outcomes. Thus, the National Institute for Dental and Craniofacial Research (NIDCR), with its focus on creating new knowledge around oral health, has particular interest in developing and testing implementation strategies that

Table 1
Dissemination and implementation definitions and examples

Term	Definition	Example
Diffusion	Diffusion of knowledge and information that occurs without concerted promotion.[43]	• Word of mouth
Dissemination	Targeted distribution of information and intervention materials to a specific public health or clinical practice audience. The intent is to spread knowledge and the associated evidence-based interventions (Implementation Science Journal).[43,44]	• Publication in peer-reviewed journal • Medical/dental society Web site (such as ebd.ada.org) • Podcast • Webinar • eLearning and live learning courses • Online repositories (guidelines.gov, Guidelines International Network [G-I-N] Library, translating research into practice (TRIP) database) • Press release/public relations campaigns
Implementation	Methods to promote the systematic uptake of clinical research findings and other evidence-based practices into routine practice and hence improve the quality and effectiveness of health care (Implementation Science Journal).[75]	• Educational outreach/Academic detailing • Use of key opinion leaders and champions • Audit and feedback • Reminders • Financial incentives • Clinical decision support systems (ie, algorithms, order sets, electronic health record reminders) • Policy changes • Patient resources (ie, decision support tools, eHealth)

identify, understand, and overcome barriers to the adoption, adaptation, integration, scale-up, and sustainability of specific evidence-based interventions, tools, policies, and guidelines as they relate to dental practice. NIDCR is also interested in developing and testing strategies to "de-implement" or reduce the use of interventions, tools, policies, and guidelines that are no longer supported by current evidence, have never been evidence-based, have been prematurely widely adopted, and/or are harmful or wasteful.[54–57]

IMPLEMENTATION OF CLINICAL PRACTICE GUIDELINES

One overarching goal of implementation science is understanding how to effectively implement CPGs such that they become routine and sustainable elements in a given clinical practice setting. Basing implementation strategies on behavior change theory tends to improve guideline adoption, but inherent factors unique to each new guideline and barriers unique within each practice setting may prevent complete adoption at either the individual provider or organizational level. As an example, in an analysis of guidelines and their specific recommendations, clear recommendations were implemented in 67% of clinical decisions, compared with only 36% of decisions when the recommendations were vague and imprecisely defined.[55] Additionally, guidelines in which lack of compliance can lead to tort action concerns (eg, guidelines for prevention of infective endocarditis) are more readily adopted than are guidelines that for many seem optional and possibly outside the standard of care (eg, the American Dental Association [ADA] dental sealant guideline recommending applying dental sealants to noncavitated occlusal caries).

Tools have been developed to support guidelines implementation. Examples of such tools include algorithms, guideline summaries, clinical decision-making tools or clinical decision support, patient communication tools, and guidance for evaluation.[56–58]

Clinical decision support (CDS) within the electronic health record (EHR) has the potential to improve the implementation of scientific evidence into clinical practice by providing relevant information to the clinician at the point of care in a concise manner that fits into the clinic workflow.[31,38,59] For example, a Cochrane review examined the use of the EHR to improve smoking cessation,[60] and concluded that an EHR using CDS could improve treatment by improving the fidelity of adherence to clinical guidelines.

IMPLEMENTATION OF CLINICAL PRACTICE GUIDELINES IN DENTISTRY

Implementation science applied to dentistry faces many challenges. First, although dental care is delivered in a variety of practice settings, including small private practices, community clinics, hospitals, and large group practices, most dental care is still delivered in small private offices. Compared with medicine, dentistry is still effectively a cottage industry, meaning that there is little external oversight of care delivery or clinical decisions made by dentists. Second, the ability to measure actual practice change is limited due to lack of standardization of data entered into the EHR. This includes the current lack of use of diagnostic codes in the EHR. The inability to link treatment to need (ie, diagnosis) is a barrier to monitoring the appropriateness of clinical practice. Adding to this is that dentists (as with most clinicians) do not think if their patients as a "population," meaning that measuring practice patterns, and patient outcomes at the aggregate level of their total patient population is rarely done. Exceptions exist to this and include large multiprovider care networks, such as the Kaiser Permanente system and to a lesser degree within the National Dental Practice-based Research Network.[61]

In these settings, there is an ability to capture patient population-level outcomes and to more accurately characterize provider behavior as it relates to fidelity to CPGs.

The NIDCR has prioritized implementation science among its extramural efforts.[62] The institute has identified parameters to consider as implementation science is embarked in dentistry: differentiating implementation research from effectiveness research, determining when clinical practices are ready for scale-up or de-implementation, identifying potential levers for practice change, and assessing existing infrastructure to support implementation research. They have acknowledged that long-standing reliance on continuing education training as a stand-alone strategy has proven to be insufficient for effecting change; rather, stressing the need for systemic, multicomponent strategies to be developed to address the multilevel contexts in which care is delivered.

In dentistry, pit-and-fissure sealants provide an illustrative example of the issues that confront effective implementation. Evidence-based guidelines have been widely available in dentistry at least since the ADA launched its Center for Evidence-based Dentistry in 2006. The ADA's guideline platform does include a number of implementation tools, the principal one being its Chairside Guides that serve as a synthesis of the key guideline recommendation to enhance their use in clinical settings. However, evaluation of the extent of guideline implementation in dentistry has been limited. What analysis has been conducted has centered around the use of pit-and-fissure sealants for primary and secondary caries prevention, and no evaluation of implementation tools in dentistry has been conducted.

The ADA published its first sealant guideline in 2008,[12] which was subsequently updated in 2016.[13] The evidence in support of pit-and-fissure sealants is supported by guidelines developed by other organizations as well.[63–67] In the ADA's case, the sealant guideline is based on several well-done systematic reviews documenting their efficacy. As a result of the large benefit derived from appropriate sealant application, the Dental Quality Alliance developed a quality of care performance measure for sealants,[68] and Healthy People 2020 includes dental sealants in their goals.[69] Taken together, the cumulative evidence and guidance available to support use of pit-and-fissure sealants, and adoption of corresponding evidence, is among the highest available for any dental preventive or therapeutic procedure. Despite this robust evidence of efficacy, adoption of the guideline's recommendations in most dental settings has been disappointing.[34,39]

Barriers preventing implementation of pit-and-fissure sealants have been assessed at the individual provider and organizational levels. Individual barriers include lack of awareness of the guidelines and the supporting evidence, and lack of awareness or ability to distinguish early lesions that may be arrested with a sealant, skepticism about the evidence of sealants for caries arrest, denial that sealants are the standard of care, and fear of the impact of residual decay in ongoing cariogenic process.[39,40,70]

Organizational barriers include lack of organizational workflow to enable leveraging sealants for primary and secondary prevention and lack of financial incentive in the current reimbursement structure.[40] Potential organizational facilitators that may enhance sealant guideline implementation include a vision toward evidence-based medicine and disease prevention supported by organizational leadership.[70]

Efforts toward implementation tools and strategies to promote sealant guideline implementation are limited. The ADA does have a robust Chairside Guide available to support this guideline.[71] An implementation strategy to promote sealant placement in the United Kingdom was developed and evaluated.[72] The strategies tested included 4 randomized study arms: (1) fee per sealant treatment; (2) education in evidence-based practice; (3) combined fee plus education; and (4) control (neither fee nor education). Although instilling the financial incentive increased sealant placement by 9.8%, education alone had no impact. Surprisingly, the combined strategy of the financial incentive and the education fared worse than financial incentive alone.

Key components identified by the NIDCR for successful implementation of sealant guidelines,[62] which can be applied to other dental guidelines, include the following:

- *Identification of* potential barriers and develop targeted strategies. If perceived personal experience serves as a barrier, implementation strategies can include monitoring and evaluating long-term outcomes in an objective way to evaluate if perception is in concordance with actual performance. User-friendly tools may alleviate complexity of written guidelines.
- Access guideline acceptability. If acceptability is a concern, strategies may include providing opportunities for hands-on experience and mentoring.
- Address patient characteristics and preferences. This has been an area of neglect in implementation science, but may serve as a useful target for implementation.
- Assess provider knowledge, support, and self-efficacy. Implementation is dependent on willingness and perceived self-ability of health care providers to change practice patterns.
- Service delivery context. Implementation occurs at the local level, and successful implementation strategies are adaptable to local individual and organizational factors.
- Stages of implementation. At the individual and organizational levels, implementation is not instantaneous. Rather, like other examples of behavior change, implementation proceeds through staged process. Considering the current stage in the process, developing appropriate strategies is needed to succeed in sustained implementation.

Sealants are just one example in dentistry of a topic in need of implementation science–derived interventions. Other topics that could be addressed using implementation strategies include Screening, Brief Intervention, and Referral to Treatment (SBIRT), rubber dam and opioids, antibiotic de-implementation for patients with prosthetic joints, and others. SBIRT is a promising behavior change approach that could be used to address problematic oral health behaviors, such as alcohol and tobacco use.[73] Rubber dam usage was examined in a National Dental Practice-based Research Network study. Rubber dam use improves patient safety and outcomes of root canal treatment, yet this study found considerable variation in use, attitudes, and beliefs about rubber dam use.

Additionally, there is benefit in understanding the need to "de-implement" certain treatments not supported by the evidence, but have been widely adopted but potentially harmful. The current opioid epidemic demonstrating harm associated with opioid use and the evidence that nonopioid analgesics are effective at managing acute postoperative pain following extractions calls for studies on how to de-implement opioids in dentistry.[74]

SUMMARY

Translating research into practice is critical to bridging the Know-Do Gap and minimizing overuse, underuse, and misuse of health care procedures. Evidence-based guidelines serve as a critical resource toward minimizing this gap, and should be sought out and routinely used as a means to scale evidence-based practice in any dental setting. Given that dissemination of dental guidelines is not sufficient to universally change practice patterns, targeted implementation strategies can be leveraged to minimize the Know-Do Gap and facilitate translation of evidence into practice. When developing effective implementation strategies in dentistry, one needs to consider barriers and facilitators that may be context specific, and may need to be addressed at the local level for each individual practice. Developing, implementing, and evaluating a robust implementation strategy will be key for dental providers to make progress in reducing the Know-Do Gap.

REFERENCES

1. Institute of Medicine. Crossing the quality chasm: a new health system for the 21st century. 2001. Available at: http://www.nationalacademies.org/hmd/~/media/Files/Report%20Files/2001/Crossing-the-Quality-Chasm/Quality%20Chasm%202001%20%20report%20brief.pdf. Accessed May 9, 2018.
2. Grol R. Successes and failures in the implementation of evidence-based guidelines for clinical practice. Med Care 2001;39(8 Suppl 2):II46–54.
3. Schuster MA, McGlynn EA, Brook RH. How good is the quality of health care in the United States? Milbank Q 1998;76(4):517–63, 509.
4. BMJ Clinical Evidence. What conclusions has clinical evidence drawn about what works, what doesn't based on randomised controlled trial evidence? Available at: http://clinicalevidence.bmj.com/x/set/static/cms/efficacy-categorisations.html. Accessed February 18, 2018.
5. Chassin MR, Galvin RW. The urgent need to improve health care quality. Institute of Medicine National Roundtable on health care quality. JAMA 1998;280(11):1000–5.
6. Coon ER, Young PC, Quinonez RA, et al. 2017 update on pediatric medical overuse: a review. JAMA Pediatr 2018;172(5):482–6.
7. Morgan DJ, Dhruva SS, Coon ER, et al. 2017 update on medical overuse: a systematic review. JAMA Intern Med 2018;178(1):110–5.
8. Morgan DJ, Wright SM, Dhruva S. Update on medical overuse. JAMA Intern Med 2015;175(1):120–4.
9. Sollecito TP, Abt E, Lockhart PB, et al. The use of prophylactic antibiotics prior to dental procedures in patients with prosthetic joints: evidence-based clinical practice guideline for dental practitioners—a report of the American Dental Association Council on Scientific Affairs. J Am Dent Assoc 2015;146(1):11–16 e18.
10. Semrad TJ, Tancredi DJ, Baldwin LM, et al. Geographic variation of racial/ethnic disparities in colorectal cancer testing among medicare enrollees. Cancer 2011;117(8):1755–63.
11. Stiela L, Soret S, Montgomery S. Geographic patterns of change over time in mammography: differences between black and white U.S. medicare enrollees. Cancer Epidemiol 2017;46:57–65.
12. Beauchamp J, Caufield PW, Crall JJ, et al. Evidence-based clinical recommendations for the use of pit-and-fissure sealants: a report of the American Dental Association Council on Scientific Affairs. J Am Dent Assoc 2008;139(3):257–68.
13. Wright JT, Crall JJ, Fontana M, et al. Evidence-based clinical practice guideline for the use of pit-and-fissure sealants: a report of the American Dental Association and the American Academy of Pediatric Dentistry. J Am Dent Assoc 2016;147(8):672–82.e12.
14. Chen X, Faviez C, Schuck S, et al. Mining patients' narratives in social media for pharmacovigilance: adverse effects and misuse of methylphenidate. Front Pharmacol 2018;9:541.

15. Benson K, Flory K, Humphreys KL, et al. Misuse of stimulant medication among college students: a comprehensive review and meta-analysis. Clin Child Fam Psychol Rev 2015;18(1):50–76.
16. Chan WL, Wood DM, Dargan PI. Significant misuse of sildenafil in London nightclubs. Subst Use Misuse 2015;50(11):1390–4.
17. Cheatle MD. Prescription opioid misuse, abuse, morbidity, and mortality: balancing effective pain management and safety. Pain Med 2015;16(Suppl 1): S3–8.
18. Cobaugh DJ, Gainor C, Gaston CL, et al. The opioid abuse and misuse epidemic: implications for pharmacists in hospitals and health systems. Am J Health Syst Pharm 2014;71(18):1539–54.
19. Garland EL, Howard MO. Opioid attentional bias and cue-elicited craving predict future risk of prescription opioid misuse among chronic pain patients. Drug Alcohol Depend 2014;144:283–7.
20. Balas EA, Boren SA. Managing clinical knowledge for health care improvement. Yearb Med Inform 2000;(1):65–70.
21. Grant J, Green L, Mason B. Basic research and health: a reassessment of the scientific basis for the support of biomedical science. Res Eval 2003;12:217–24.
22. Glasziou P, Haynes B. The paths from research to improved health outcomes. Evid Based Nurs 2005;8(2):36–8.
23. Shaneyfelt TM. Building bridges to quality. JAMA 2001;286(20):2600–1.
24. Sackett DL, Rosenberg WM, Gray JA, et al. Evidence based medicine: what it is and what it isn't. BMJ 1996;312(7023):71–2.
25. Guyatt GH. Evidence-based medicine. ACP J Club 1991;114. A–16.
26. Smith R, Rennie D. Evidence-based medicine–an oral history. JAMA 2014;311(4): 365–7.
27. Grimshaw JM, Schunemann HJ, Burgers J, et al. Disseminating and implementing guidelines: article 13 in integrating and coordinating efforts in COPD guideline development. An official ATS/ERS workshop report. Proc Am Thorac Soc 2012;9(5):298–303.
28. Khoury MJ, Gwinn M, Ioannidis JP. The emergence of translational epidemiology: from scientific discovery to population health impact. Am J Epidemiol 2010; 172(5):517–24.
29. Field MJ, Lohr KN, editors. Clinical practice guidelines: directions for a new program. Washington, DC: National Academies Press; 1990.
30. Pronovost PJ. Enhancing physicians' use of clinical guidelines. JAMA 2013; 310(23):2501–2.
31. van Wijk MA, van der Lei J, Mosseveld M, et al. Compliance of general practitioners with a guideline-based decision support system for ordering blood tests. Clin Chem 2002;48(1):55–60.
32. Grimshaw JM, Russell IT. Effect of clinical guidelines on medical practice: a systematic review of rigorous evaluations. Lancet 1993;342(8883):1317–22.
33. Armstrong JJ, Goldfarb AM, Instrum RS, et al. Improvement evident but still necessary in clinical practice guideline quality: a systematic review. J Clin Epidemiol 2017;81:13–21.
34. Tellez M, Gray SL, Gray S, et al. Sealants and dental caries: dentists' perspectives on evidence-based recommendations. J Am Dent Assoc 2011;142(9): 1033–40.
35. Weisz G, Cambrosio A, Keating P, et al. The emergence of clinical practice guidelines. Milbank Q 2007;85(4):691–727.

36. Davis DA, Taylor-Vaisey A. Translating guidelines into practice. A systematic review of theoretic concepts, practical experience and research evidence in the adoption of clinical practice guidelines. CMAJ 1997;157(4):408–16.
37. Shekelle PG, Ortiz E, Rhodes S, et al. Validity of the agency for healthcare research and quality clinical practice guidelines: how quickly do guidelines become outdated? JAMA 2001;286(12):1461–7.
38. Bero LA, Grilli R, Grimshaw JM, et al. Closing the gap between research and practice: an overview of systematic reviews of interventions to promote the implementation of research findings. The Cochrane effective practice and Organization of Care Review Group. BMJ 1998;317(7156):465–8.
39. O'Donnell JA, Modesto A, Oakley M, et al. Sealants and dental caries: insight into dentists' behaviors regarding implementation of clinical practice recommendations. J Am Dent Assoc 2013;144(4):e24–30.
40. Spallek H, Song M, Polk DE, et al. Barriers to implementing evidence-based clinical guidelines: a survey of early adopters. J Evid Based Dent Pract 2010;10(4):195–206.
41. Leach CW, van Zomeren M, Zebel S, et al. Group-level self-definition and self-investment: a hierarchical (multicomponent) model of in-group identification. J Pers Soc Psychol 2008;95(1):144–65.
42. Implementation Science. Aims and scope. Available at: http://www.imple mentationscience.com/about#aimsscope. Accessed February 18, 2018.
43. Rogers EM. Diffusion of innovations. 5th edition. New York: Free Press; 2003.
44. US Dept of Health and Human Services. Program announcement number PAR-10-038. Available at: http://grants.nih.gov/grants/guide/pa-files/PAR-10- 038. html. Accessed February 18, 2018.
45. Brownson RC, Chriqui JF, Stamatakis KA. Understanding evidence-based public health policy. Am J Public Health 2009;99(9):1576–83.
46. Glisson C, Schoenwald SK, Hemmelgarn A, et al. Randomized trial of MST and ARC in a two-level evidence-based treatment implementation strategy. J Consult Clin Psychol 2010;78(4):537–50.
47. Ruhe MC, Weyer SM, Zronek S, et al. Facilitating practice change: lessons from the STEP-UP clinical trial. Prev Med 2005;40(6):729–34.
48. Glasgow RE, Vinson C, Chambers D, et al. National Institutes of Health approaches to dissemination and implementation science: current and future directions. Am J Public Health 2012;102(7):1274–81.
49. Greenhalgh T, Robert G, MacFarlane F, et al. Diffusion of innovations in service organizations: systematic review and recommendations. Milbank Q 2004;82(4):581–629.
50. Oxman A, Flottorp S. An overview of strategies to promote implementation of evidence-based health care. In: Silagy C, Haines A, editors. Evidence-based practice in primary care. 2nd edition. London: BMJ books; 2001.
51. Cabana MD, Rand CS, Powe NR, et al. Why don't physicians follow clinical practice guidelines? A framework for improvement. JAMA 1999;282(15):1458–65.
52. Grol R. Personal paper. Beliefs and evidence in changing clinical practice. BMJ 1997;315(7105):418–21.
53. Haines A, Rogers S. Integrating research evidence into practice. In: Silagy C, Haines A, editors. Evidence-based practice in primary care. 2nd edition. London: BMJ books; 2001.
54. National Institute of Dental and Craniofacial Research. Behavioral & social sciences research program. Available at: https://www.nidcr.nih.gov/grants-funding/

grant-programs/behavioral-social-sciences-research-program/more.   Accessed May 11, 2018.

55. Grol R, Dalhuijsen J, Thomas S, et al. Attributes of clinical guidelines that influence use of guidelines in general practice: observational study. BMJ 1998; 317(7162):858–61.

56. Dobbins M, Hanna SE, Ciliska D, et al. A randomized controlled trial evaluating the impact of knowledge translation and exchange strategies. Implement Sci 2009;4:61.

57. McKillop A, Crisp J, Walsh K. Practice guidelines need to address the 'how' and the 'what' of implementation. Prim Health Care Res Dev 2012;13(1):48–59.

58. Shekelle PG, Kravitz RL, Beart J, et al. Are nonspecific practice guidelines potentially harmful? A randomized comparison of the effect of nonspecific versus specific guidelines on physician decision making. Health Serv Res 2000;34(7): 1429–48.

59. Hillestad R, Bigelow J, Bower A, et al. Can electronic medical record systems transform health care? Potential health benefits, savings, and costs. Health Aff (Millwood) 2005;24(5):1103–17.

60. Boyle R, Solberg L, Fiore M. Use of electronic health records to support smoking cessation. Cochrane Database Syst Rev 2011;(12):CD008743.

61. The National Dental Practice-based Research Network. Leveraging electronic dental record data for clinical research. Available at: http://www.nationaldentalpbrn.org/leveraging-electronic-dental-record-data-for-clinical-research.php. Accessed May 11, 2018.

62. Clark DB, Ducharme L. Charting a course for implementation research in oral health. JDR Clin Trans Res 2016;9(3):198–200.

63. Gooch BF, Griffin SO, Gray SK, et al. Preventing dental caries through school-based sealant programs: updated recommendations and reviews of evidence. J Am Dent Assoc 2009;140(11):1356–65.

64. Oral Health Services Research Centre. Pit and fissure sealants: evidence-based guidance on the use of sealants for the prevention and management of pit and fissure caries. Cork (Ireland): Oral Health Services Research Centre; 2010.

65. Scottish Intercollegiate Guidelines Network. Dental interventions to prevent caries in children. A national clinical guideline. Edinburgh (Scotland): Scottish Intercollegiate Guideline Network; 2014.

66. American Academy of Pediatric Dentistry. Guideline on caries-risk assessment and management for infants, children, and adolescents. Chicago: American Academy of Pediatric Dentistry; 2011.

67. Community Preventive Services Task Force. Oral health: preventing dental caries, school-based dental sealant delivery programs. 2013. Available at: https://www.thecommunityguide.org/sites/default/files/assets/Oral-Health-Caries-School-based-Sealants_0.pdf. Accessed September 5, 2018.

68. American Dental Association Dental Quality Alliance. Oral health sealant for children between 6-9 years. 2014. Available at: https://ushik.ahrq.gov/ViewItemDetails?&system=dcqm&itemKey=202157000&enableAsynchronousLoading=true.   Accessed February 12, 2017.

69. Office of Disease Prevention and Health Promotion. Healthy People 2020. Oral Health. Available at: https://www.healthypeople.gov/2020/topics-objectives/topic/oral-health/objectives. Accessed May 11, 2018.

70. Polk DE, Weyant RJ, Shah NH, et al. Barriers to sealant guideline implementation within a multi-site managed care dental practice. BMC Oral Health 2018;18(1):17.

71. Dentistry ADACfE-B. Evidence-based clinical practice guideline for the use of pit-and-fissure sealants: chairside guide. Available at: https://ebd.ada.org/~/media/EBD/Files/ADA-AAPD_2016_Guide_Sealants.pdf?la=en. Accessed May 11, 2018.

72. Clarkson JE, Turner S, Grimshaw JM, et al. Changing clinicians' behavior: a randomized controlled trial of fees and education. J Dent Res 2008;87(7):640–4.

73. Cuevas J, Chi DL. SBIRT-based interventions to improve pediatric oral health behaviors and outcomes: considerations for future behavioral SBIRT interventions in dentistry. Curr Oral Health Rep 2016;3(3):187–92.

74. Moore PA, Ziegler KM, Lipman RD, et al. Benefits and harms associated with analgesic medications used in the management of acute dental pain: an overview of systematic reviews. J Am Dent Assoc 2018;149(4):256–265 e3.

75. Available at: https://implementationscience.biomedcentral.com/about. Accessed September 5, 2018.

How Should We Evaluate and Use Evidence to Improve Population Oral Health?

Paul R. Brocklehurst, BDS, MDPH, PhD, FFGDP, FDS RCS (Eng)[a],*,
Sarah R. Baker, BSc, PhD, AFBPsS[b], Stefan Listl, DDS, PhD[c],
Marco A. Peres, BDS, MSc, PhD[d], Georgios Tsakos, BDS, MSc, PhD, FHEA[e],
Jo Rycroft-Malone, RN, MSc, PhD[f]

KEYWORDS

- Population health • Public health • Implementation • Evidence-based dentistry

KEY POINTS

- This article questions an uncritical adoption of the evidence-based paradigm for interventions to improve oral health at a population level.
- A linear logic model that links the generation of research evidence with its use is overly simplistic.
- This article explores approaches to the evaluation of complex interventions in dentistry and how they can be embedded into policy and practice.

BACKGROUND

Half of the world's population suffers from untreated oral conditions, affecting a total of 3.5 billion people in 2015; 2.5 billion people were affected by untreated caries in permanent teeth, 573 million children by untreated caries in deciduous teeth, 538 million people by severe periodontal disease, and 276 million people were affected by total tooth loss.[1] Dental diseases produce large societal costs, both in terms of treatment costs and losses to productivity; for the twenty-eight countries in the European Union,

Disclosure Statement: The authors have nothing to declare.
Financial Disclosure: There are no known commercial or financial conflicts of interest or funding sources for any of the authors.
[a] Normal Site, Bangor University, Bangor, UK; [b] The School of Clinical Dentistry, University of Sheffield, Sheffield, UK; [c] Faculty of Medical Sciences, Radboud University, The Netherlands; [d] Adelaide Dental School, The University of Adelaide, Adelaide, South Australia, Australia; [e] Department of Epidemiology and Public Health, University College, 1-19 Torrington Place, London, UK; [f] Main Arts Building, Bangor University, Bangor, UK
* Corresponding author.
E-mail address: p.brocklehurst@bangor.ac.uk

dental.theclinics.com

dental diseases led to treatment costs of $100 billion (€92 billion) and productivity losses of $57 billion (€52 billion) in 2015.[2,3]

Given this, generating and implementing evidence-based policy are important aims for many publicly funded health systems.[4] In dentistry, this is based on the assumption that evidence-based health care increases the efficiency and effectiveness of interventions to improve oral health at a population level.[5] It is increasingly recognized, however, that a linear or logic model that links the generation of research evidence with its use is overly simplistic.[6] This article challenges an uncritical interpretation of the evidence-based paradigm and explores approaches to the evaluation of complex interventions and how they can be embedded into policy and practice to improve oral health at a population level.

THE CHALLENGE OF GENERATING THE EVIDENCE

The process of generating robust research evidence has traditionally relied on randomized controlled clinical trials (RCTs) to empirically evaluate interventions.[7] Any observed effect is pooled statistically and the evidence is then synthesized to create evidence-based policies.[8] Research evidence is then either pushed from the research community (in guidelines or evidence summaries) or pulled by clinicians who are seeking evidence-based approaches to inform their approach to care. There are several inherent difficulties, however, with a push-pull assumption when the intervention is complex[9] or where it attempts to "introduce new, or modify existing, patterns of collective action in health care or some other formal organisational setting."[10,11]

The first problem is that the quality of many trials remains poor. In Glasziou and colleagues'[12] study, 40% to 89% of the interventions were not replicable due to a poor description and, in most studies, at least 1 primary outcome measure was changed, introduced, or omitted. In Yordanov and colleagues'[13] methodological review and simulation study of trials included in Cochrane reviews, 43% of the 1286 studies identified had at least 1 domain at high risk of bias and 142 of a random sample of 200 of the aforementioned trials were confirmed as high risk. Secondly, "trialists routinely claim that uncertainty doesn't exist. We pick single point estimates for all of these parameters, create a design that would work well if all of those guesses happen to be true simultaneously (a very unlikely event) and then we put that design into a grant that we hope gets funded'.[14] As further highlighted by Lewis,[14] "this approach leads to an increased risk of falsely negative or inconclusive results."

An even more fundamental issue is that effect sizes alone are not enough to facilitate the implementation of research findings in clinical practice or public health: "effect sizes do not provide policy makers with information on how an intervention might be replicated in their specific context, or whether trial outcomes will be reproduced."[15] As Grant and colleagues[16] highlight, one of the reasons why so much clinical research is ignored is because "there is not enough contextual information provided to transfer the results from the trial setting into other settings." A further problem is the common conflation of efficacy and effectiveness; demonstrating that a health technology works (efficacy) does not necessarily mean that it can improve health at a population level (effectiveness).[17]

Another critique of the evidence-based paradigm relates to how evidence is synthesized and analyzed. Trials with positive results are published in approximately 4 years to 5 years, whereas trials with null or negative results take 6 years to 8 years to publish.[18] Because multiple trials are required for 1 systematic review, they become highly resource intensive.[19] This contrasts with the often rapidly moving policy context where structures at microlevel, mesolevel, and macrolevel (ie, at the levels of the clinician, commissioner of services, and governments, respectively) can change quickly. As Gannan and colleagues[20] highlight, "emerging issues require access to high-quality evidence in a timely manner to inform system and policy response."

Another concern with the process is that many systematic review methodologies have a tendency to strip out the policy context. This has led some researchers to adopt a theoretic approach to help guide the process of the review and make sure key elements are retained, particularly where the intervention is complex. Implementation frameworks, such as the Knowledge to Action framework,[21] and other methods (for example, realist syntheses) explicitly seek to include and understand the role of context and how and why interventions or programs work.[22] The authors consider this critical. As Northridge and Metcalf highlight, there is a "need to extract the core issues from the context in which they are embedded in order to better ensure that they are transferable across settings."[23] Such insights highlight the value of shifting from the traditionally used binary question of effectiveness toward a more sophisticated explanation.[24]

Once evidence has been synthesized, the response by the evidence user can be idiosyncratic and these problems become magnified when interventions are introduced into complex social or organizational systems.[25] Several system-related challenges relate to this process and introduce variation that needs to be considered and managed. Such challenges refer to the variability and stability (and predictability) across and within organizations, the range of solutions applicable to any given problem, the multiple mechanisms involved, the differing ability of the individual/organization to affect these mechanisms, and the varying relationships between mechanisms and outcomes (in terms of linearity and impact).[26] Equally, evidence is often weighed alongside other clinical factors and experiential knowledge can be privileged.[27,28] As a result, the production of evidence in its own right is not sufficient per se to influence change.[29] Decision making is a process, not a one-off event, and relies on productive ongoing relationships and the organizational context.[30,31]

PRODUCING CHANGE IN POPULATION ORAL HEALTH?

One of the key challenges relates to the relevance of the RCTs and the degree of their use to shape policy aiming to improve a population's oral health. There is evidence that outputs from trials have had a direct impact on public health policy. Recently, Chestnutt and colleagues'[32] Seal or Varnish? trial led to a near immediate cessation of a national sealant scheme across Wales in favor of a fluoride varnish scheme. They concluded that "in a community oral health programme utilising mobile dental clinics and targeted at children with high caries risk, the twice-yearly application of fluoride varnish resulted in caries prevention that is not significantly different from that obtained by applying and maintaining fissure sealants after 36 months" and that fluoride varnish was more cost effective. Equally, Milsom and colleagues'[33] trial on dental screening programs for school-aged children produced a policy change by the National Screening Committee in the United Kingdom and Innes and colleagues's[34] trial on the Hall technique made a substantive impact on the management of child caries. This is in contrast, however, with several trials whose results have had less impact to date.[35,36]

As highlighted previously, the use of the evidence-based paradigm can be applied without critical thought. At a population level, there are arguments for the inclusion of other study designs to augment the evaluation of dental public health programs and health policies.[37] The recent debate after the publication of the Cochrane review on the effectiveness of water fluoridation illustrates this point. This review was influenced by the exclusion of observational studies and concluded that "there is very little contemporary evidence, meeting the review's inclusion criteria."[38] In their critique, however, Rugg-Gunn and colleagues[39] argued that "with public health interventions....there are frequently no such trials because the highly complex practical, ethical and financial factors involved mean that RCTs are not feasible." They go on to argue that unlike individual clinical interventions, evidence has to be drawn from a wide variety of research designs to determine whether a complex public health intervention is cost effective. This approach was undertaken by the National Health and Medical Research Center (NHMRC) in Australia, which reached a different conclusion: "the NHMRC strongly recommends community water fluoridation as a safe, effective and ethical way to help reduce tooth decay across the population."[40]

Antibiotic prophylaxis for infective endocarditis is another example. This was common-place in the UK until 2008, when the National Institute of Care Excellence (NICE) stated that "antibiotic prophylaxis against infective endocarditis is *not recommended* for people undergoing dental procedures."[41] NICE relies heavily on evidence from clinical trials and evidence from other study designs downgraded; as such, it seemed locked into a recommendation that was at odds with the international consensus.[42] It also became at odds with a large observational study that demonstrated that the cessation of antibiotic prophylaxis (NICE guidance) had increased the risk of patients contracting infective endocarditis.[43] In recognition of this confusion and yet without any further evidence, NICE changed its recommendation in 2016 to "antibiotic prophylaxis against infective endocarditis is not recommended routinely for people undergoing dental procedures," creating a great deal of confusion.[44]

The use of taxation for sugar-sweetened beverages (SSBs) is another area where the uncritical adoption of the evidence-based paradigm is problematic. Empirically evaluating the impact of a sugar tax would require participants to be randomized to different price levels in any 1 country. This is unfeasible. Furthermore, making cross-country comparisons would be highly resource intensive and a systematic review using multiple trials even more unlikely.

Quasi-experimental methodologies have been used to show reduction in the consumption of SSBs and an increase in water consumption after implementing a sugar tax,[45] while modeling studies have explored the potential impact of such an intervention on population health and the economy.[46] In the absence of evidence from experimental evidence, a health care decision maker has to ask, Which other types of information are suitable for timely and evidence-informed decision making? Health policies, particularly with regard to public health, often need to be formulated at a time point when the respective evidence base is still limited.[47] And the traditional evidence-based model around RCTs does not fit well public health interventions that require strong theoretic underpinnings, wider methodological approaches, and a focus on complex systems.[48]

THE APPLICATION OF THEORETIC APPROACHES TO HELP EVIDENCE USE

Psychological theory is increasingly used to predict individual behavior change and improve the adoption of evidence.[49] These theories set out to understand the proximal determinants of behavior including beliefs (cognitions), knowledge, and the attitudes and motivations that underlie an individual's behavioral intentions and ultimately behavior.[50,51] The underlying assumption is that understanding behavior is enough to produce changes at scale.[52] Such approaches have been used in dentistry in relation to adherence to guidelines for fissure sealants,[53] intraoral radiographs,[54] caries management for children,[55] and advising on oral health–related behaviors.[56]

To date, psychological theories have been shown to be important because they target behavioral drivers that are potentially amenable to change.[57] Recent developments have also seen an attempt to synthesize these. The Theoretical Domains Framework (TDF) brings together a large number of psychological theories and constructs that have been found to influence health professionals' behavior.[58,59] The 14 domains of the TDF include constructs, such as knowledge, skills, social/professional role and identity, and beliefs about capability.[60]

The TDF has also been applied to dentistry: antibiotic prescribing,[61] caries management,[62,63] and the application of fluoride varnish to children's teeth.[64] There remains a lack of focus, however, on the organizational context, including practice culture and other factors that can influence individual clinician decision making. This is problematic because the implementation of evidence requires complex changes in clinical practice within complex health systems. These take place not because of individual behavioral processes but through collective action enacted by teams within health care organisations.[65] For example, dentists do not adopt evidence-based preventive care because of a lack of inertia or up-to-date knowledge or skills but commonly because of practical (existing logistics of the dental practice), cultural (dentists' perceptions of their patients and patient motivations, values, and cooperativeness), and economic (time constraints, financial risk, and funding systems) barriers.[66,67] Arguably, rather than targeting different levels for effective change—individual clinician (eg, dentist and dental hygienist), health care unit or team (eg, dental practice), or health care organization (eg, National Health Service)—the system as a whole needs to be considered.[68]

WHAT CAN IMPLEMENTATION SCIENCE OFFER?

Given the persistent and often intractable challenges of evidence-based health care, there has been a growing interest in the study of implementation processes and approaches to unpack the black box. Implementation research reinforces the assertion that evidence production does not naturally flow into evidence use. As discussed previously, people use tacit and collective knowledge to determine whether evidence is credible and whether it fits with their experience and practice.[28] Evidence users are not passive recipients and their practice is influenced by the context in which they work. Organization features, such as organizational slack, resources, the nature and quality of leadership, culture, and communication systems, are all important.[69]

The evidence base suggests that there is more promise in approaches that are theoretically based, interactive, and tailored.[70] For example, there is growing support for the use of change agents in implementation processes. One such change agent is facilitation, where evidence is 3 times more likely to be adopted.[71,72] Training lay workers as facilitators of quality improvement in Vietnam showed a significantly positive effect on neonatal mortality.[73] Implementation frameworks are also important in the choice and development of interventions, for identifying appropriate outcomes, measures, and variables of interest and in guiding the evaluation of implementation processes and outcomes. These include the Promoting Action on Implementation in Health Services, Knowledge to Action, the Consolidated Framework for Implementation Research, and normalization process theory. These frameworks help shift thinking away from viewing the gap between evidence and practice as being a service problem to one that acknowledges the importance of how knowledge is created. The idea that users and producers of evidence occupy 2 separate worlds has not been helpful in accelerating progress with the evidence-based practice agenda. As such, there is increasing interest in the development of more collaborative-type arrangements, such as Collaborations for Leadership in Applied Health and Care in the United Kingdom. Here, the producers and users of evidence work together to create knowledge that solve service challenges in more coproductive ways.

DISCUSSION

This article argues that an uncritical adherence to the evidence-based paradigm is not always feasible, desirable, or ethical for complex health care interventions.[74] In addition, it argues that evidence production is not enough to stimulate evidence use, particularly highlighting the importance of carefully considering the theoretic underpinnings of change and the role of the context for implementation.

There are several pragmatic steps that could be taken when designing trials of complex interventions to approve adoption. These include thinking about implementation a priori and working with policy makers, commissioners, public health officials, clinicians, and the public at the beginning of the evidence generation process to ensure that the research agenda is coproduced. Factors associated with the context of a complex intervention should also be considered at the earliest stage in the evaluation process, using theoretically informed feasibility and pilot studies.[75] Theoretic frameworks should be used more prospectively as part of the trial design process for complex interventions (or other ex post methodologies).[76,77] Equally, process evaluations should be run in parallel alongside empirical evaluations of complex interventions to help understand "the causal assumptions underpinning the intervention and…how interventions work in practice."[15] In addition, the use of Studies Within A Trial can help understand the best way to ensure adequate representation of those that are recruited.[78]

The standardization of outcome measures used in trials of amenable population programs to promote oral health would also be of real value. As highlighted by Kirkham and colleagues,[79] there is "growing recognition that insufficient attention has been paid to the outcomes measured in clinical trials, which need to be relevant to health service users and other people making choices about health care if the findings of research are to influence practice." In the past, the heterogeneity of outcome measures used by many trialists has made meta-analysis difficult and has added to research waste. By taking a coproduced approach to developing a core outcome set, this type of research waste can be reduced.[78] This heterogeneity of outcomes measurement has also been a feature of oral health research and work to validate core outcome sets (eg, the current project between the World Dental Federation and the International Consortium for Health Outcomes Measurement) may inform the consistent selection of oral health outcomes for relevant interventions.

More thought should be given to the type of evidence that is assimilated in systematic reviews of large-scale programs to improve oral health, including the use of ex post and ex ante designs. Ex post techniques typically evaluate the impact of an already implemented health policy program and include a range of quasiexperimental methods, including instrumental variables, difference-in-difference, panel data analyses using fixed or random effects, and regression discontinuity designs (see Listl and colleagues[80]). A recent study used such an approach to evaluate the impact of an SSB tax in Mexico. The study showed a significant reduction in consumption since its introduction in 2014.[81] In contrast, ex ante techniques are designed to simulate the future response resulting from hypothetical interventions and to make comparisons with simulated alternative scenarios of interest to the decision maker.[73] Ex ante methods include structural modeling, agent-based modeling, and microsimulation and unlike the ex post methods can help predict the short-term, mid-term, and long-term health effects of an intervention.[82,83] Such methodologies can provide helpful information on the evaluation of policies and interventions that otherwise would not be rigorously evaluated as the standard RCT-related methodologies are neither feasible nor suitable.

More attention should be paid to an understanding of context and attempts should be made to not throw away evidence during the assimilation process that could help describe pathway to impact. Again, the use of theoretic frameworks and logic models to help guide the review process is key.[84] Such approaches can "aid in the conceptualization of the review focus and illustrate hypothesized causal links, identify effect mediators or moderators, specify intermediate outcomes and potential harms, and justify a priori subgroup analyses when differential effects are anticipated."[85] They can describe the system into which the intervention and context takes place (system-based logic model) or the processes and causal pathways that lead to the outcomes (process-orientated logic model).[85] They can also help identify the most relevant inclusion criteria and clarify the interpretation of results for policy-relevant conclusions.

Finally, more thought should be given to the use of realist reviews and rapid realist reviews in the dental literature, which specifically account for context and try to understand the underlying program theories (what works for whom, why, and in what circumstances). These would help to provide a more nuanced understanding and augment and broaden a triangulation process with existing evidence-based approaches for large-scale change in population oral health.[86] Moving toward these suggestions presents a major but welcome challenge for oral health research because it would enrich the evaluation methodological scope and facilitate the wider use and implementation of appropriate evidence into clinical practice and public health, thereby having potential for improving the oral health of the population.

REFERENCES

1. Kassebaum NJ, Smith AG, Bernabé E, et al. Global, regional, and national prevalence, incidence, and disability-adjusted life years for oral conditions for 195 countries, 1990–2015: a systematic analysis for the global burden of diseases, injuries, and risk factors. J Dent Res 2017;96(4):380–7.
2. Listl S, Galloway J, Mossey PA, et al. Global economic impact of dental diseases. J Dent Res 2015;94(10):1355–61.
3. Righolt AJ, Jevdjevic M, Marcenes W, et al. Global-, regional-, and country-level economic impacts of dental diseases in 2015. J Dent Res 2018;97(5):501–7.
4. Greyson DL, Cunningham C, Morgan S. Information behaviour of Canadian pharmaceutical policy makers. Health Info Libr J 2012;29:16–27.
5. Zardo P, Collie A. Type, frequency and purpose of information used to inform public health policy and program decision-making. BMC Public Health 2015; 15:381.
6. Greenhalgh T, Fahy N. Research impact in the community-based health sciences: an analysis of 162 case studies from the 2014 UK research excellence framework. BMC Med 2015;13:232.
7. Sackett DL, Rosenberg WMC, Gray JAM, et al. Evidence based medicine: what it is and what it isn't. BMJ 1996;312. https://doi.org/10.1136/bmj.312.7023.71.
8. Innes NPT, Schwendicke F, Lamont T. How do we create, and improve, the evidence base? Br Dent J 2016;220:651–5.
9. Davies HTO, Powell AE, Nutley SM. Mobilising knowledge to improve UK health care: learning from other countries and other sectors - a multi-method mapping study. Health Serv Deliv Res 2015;3.

10. May C, Finch T, Mair F, et al. Understanding the implementation of complex interventions in health care: the normalization process model. BMC Health Serv Res 2007;7:148.

11. Campbell M, Fitzpatrick R, Haines A, et al. Framework for design and evaluation of complex interventions to improve health. BMJ 2000;321(7262):694–6.

12. Glasziou P, Altman DG, Bossuyt P, et al. Reducing waste from incomplete or unusable reports of biomedical research. Lancet 2014;383(9913):267–76.

13. Yordanov Y, Dechartres A, Porcher R, et al. Avoidable waste of research related to inadequate methods in clinical trials. BMJ 2015;24(350):h809.

14. Lewis RJ. The pragmatic clinical trial in a learning health care system. Clin Trials 2016;13(5):484–92.

15. Moore GF, Audrey S, Barker M, et al. Process evaluation of complex interventions: Medical Research Council guidance. BMJ 2015;350:h1258.

16. Grant A, Treweek S, Wells M. Why is so much clinical research ignored and what can we do about it? Br J Hosp Med 2016;77(Supplement 10):554–5.

17. Barratt H, Campbell M, Moore L, et al. Randomised controlled trials of complex interventions and large-scale transformation of services. Health Serv Deliv Res 2016;4:19–36.

18. Hopewell S, Clarke MJ, Stewart L, et al. Time to publication for results of clinical trials. Cochrane Database Syst Rev 2007;(2). MR000011.

19. Lehoux P, Tailliez S, Denis JL, et al. Redefining health technology assessment in Canada: diversification of products and contextualization of findings. Int J Technol Assess Health Care 2004;20:325–36.

20. Ganann R, Ciliska D, Thomas H. Expediting systematic reviews: methods and implications of rapid reviews. Implement Sci 2010;5:56.

21. Graham I, Logan J, Harrison M, et al. Lost in knowledge translation: time for a map? J Contin Educ Health Prof 2006;26:13–24.

22. Wong G, Greenhalgh T, Westhorp G, et al. RAMESES publication standards: realist syntheses. BMC Med 2013;11(21). https://doi.org/10.1186/1741-7015-11-21.

23. Northridge ME, Metcalf SS. Enhancing implementation science by applying best principles of systems science. Health Res Policy Syst 2016;14:74.

24. Bate P, Robert G, Fulop N, et al. Perspectives on context. London (United Kingdom): The Health Foundation; 2014.

25. Greenhalgh T, Wieringa S. Is it time to drop the 'knowledge translation' metaphor? A critical literature review. J R Soc Med 2011;104:501–9.

26. Snowden D. Cynefin: a sense of time and space, the social ecology of knowledge management. In: Despres C, Chauvel D, editors. Knowledge horizons: the present and the promise of knowledge management. Boston: Butterworth-Heinemann; 2000. p. 344.

27. Rycroft-Malone J, Harvey G, Seers K, et al. An exploration of the factors that influence the implementation of evidence into practice. J Clin Nurs 2004;13(8):913–24.

28. Dopson S, FitzGerald L, Ferlie E, et al. No magic targets! Changing clinical practice to become more evidence based. Health Care Manage Rev 2002;27:35–47.

29. Rycroft-Malone J, Burton CR, Wilkinson J, et al. Collective action for implementation: a realist evaluation of organisational collaboration in healthcare. Implement Sci 2016;11:17.

30. Currie G, Waring J, Finn R. The limits of knowledge management for UK public services modernization: the case of patient safety and service quality. Pub Admin 2008;86(2):363–85.

31. Salter KL, Kothari A. Knowledge 'Translation' as social learning: negotiating the uptake of research-based knowledge in practice. BMC Med Educ 2016;16:76.
32. Chestnutt IG, Hutchings S, Playle S, et al. Seal or Varnish? A randomised controlled trial to determine the relative cost and effectiveness of pit and fissure sealant and fluoride varnish in preventing dental decay. Health Tech Assess 2017;21(21):1–256.
33. Milsom K, Blinkhorn A, Worthington H, et al. The effectiveness of school dental screening: a cluster-randomized control trial. J Dent Res 2006;85(10):924–8.
34. Innes NP, Evans DJ, Stirrups DR. The Hall Technique; a randomized controlled clinical trial of a novel method of managing carious primary molars in general dental practice: acceptability of the technique and outcomes at 23 months. BMC Oral Health 2007;7:18.
35. Tickle M, O'Neill C, Donaldson M, et al. A randomised controlled trial to measure the effects and costs of a dental caries prevention regime for young children attending primary care dental services: the Northern Ireland Caries Prevention In Practice (NIC-PIP) trial. Health Tech Assess 2016;20(71):1–96.
36. Milsom KM, Blinkhorn AS, Walsh T, et al. A cluster-randomized controlled trial: fluoride varnish in school children. J Dent Res 2011;90(11):1306–11.
37. Victora CG, Habicht JP, Bryce J. Evidence-based public health: moving beyond randomized trials. Am J Public Health 2004;94(3):400–5.
38. Iheozor-Ejiofor Z, Worthington HV, Walsh T, et al. Water fluoridation for the prevention of dental caries. Cochrane Database Syst Rev 2015;(6):CD010856.
39. Rugg-Gunn AJ, Spencer AJ, Whelton HP, et al. Critique of the review of 'Water fluoridation for the prevention of dental caries' published by the Cochrane Collaboration in 2015. Br Dent J 2016;220:335–40.
40. National Health and Medical Research Council (NHMRC). Information paper – water fluoridation: dental and other human health outcomes. report prepared by the Clinical Trials Centre at University of Sydney. Canberra (Australia): NHMRC; 2017.
41. Thornhill MH, Dayer M, Lockhart PB, et al. Guidelines on prophylaxis to prevent infective endocarditis. Br Dent J 2016;220:51–6.
42. Habib G, Hoen B, Tornos P, et al. Guidelines on the prevention, diagnosis, and treatment of infective endocarditis (new version 2009): the Task Force on the Prevention, Diagnosis, and Treatment of Infective Endocarditis of the European Society of Cardiology (ESC). Endorsed by the European Society of Clinical Microbiology and Infectious Diseases (ESCMID) and the International Society of Chemotherapy (ISC) for Infection and Cancer. Eur Heart J 2009;30:2369–413.
43. Dayer MJ, Jones S, Prendergast B, et al. Incidence of infective endocarditis in England, 2000–13: a secular trend, interrupted time-series analysis. Lancet 2015;385:1219–28.
44. Thornhill MH, Dayer M, Lockhart PB, et al. A change in the NICE guidelines on antibiotic prophylaxis. Br Dent J 2016;221:112–4.
45. Colchero MA, Molina M, Guerrero-López CM. After Mexico implemented a tax, purchases of sugar-sweetened beverages decreased and water increased: difference by place of residence, household composition, and income level. J Nutr 2017;147(8):1552–7.
46. Briggs ADM, Mytton OT, Kehlbacher A, et al. Health impact assessment of the UK soft drinks industry levy: a comparative risk assessment modelling study. Lancet Public Health 2017;2(1):e15–22.
47. Zucchelli E, Jones AM, Rice N. The evaluation of health policies through dynamic microsimulation methods. Int J Microsim 2012;5(1):2–20.

48. Rutter H, Savona N, Glonti K, et al. The need for a complex systems model of evidence for public health. Lancet 2017;390:2602–4.

49. Eccles MP, Grimshaw J, Walker A, et al. Changing the behaviour of healthcare professionals: the use of theory in promoting the uptake of research findings. J Clin Epidemiol 2005;58:107–12.

50. Eccles MP, Grimshaw JM, MacLennan G, et al. Explaining clinical behaviours using multiple theoretical models. Implement Sci 2012;7:99.

51. Godin G, Belanger-Gravel A, Eccles M, et al. Healthcare professionals' intentions and behaviours: a systematic review of studies based on social cognitive theories. Implement Sci 2008;3:36.

52. Michie S, Fixsen D, Grimshaw JM, et al. Specifying and reporting complex behaviour change interventions: the need for a scientific method. Implement Sci 2009;4. https://doi.org/10.1186/1748-5908-1184-1140.

53. Bonetti D, Johnston M, Clarkson J, et al. Applying psychological theories to evidence-based clinical practice: identifying factors predictive of placing fissure sealants. Implement Sci 2010;5:25.

54. Bonetti DL, Pitts N, Eccles M, et al. Applying psychological theory to evidence-based clinical practice: identifying factors predictive of taking intra-oral radiographs. Soc Sci Med 2006;63:1889–99.

55. Bonetti DL, Johnston M, Turner S, et al. Applying multiple models to predict clinicians' behavioural intention and objective behaviour when managing children's teeth. Psychol Health 2009;24:843–60.

56. Yusuf H, Kolliakou A, Ntouva A, et al. Predictors of dentists' behaviours in delivering prevention in primary dental care in England: using the theory of planned behaviour. Br Dent J 2016;16:44.

57. Asimakopoulou K, Newton JT. The contributions of behaviour change science towards dental public health practice: a new paradigm. Community Dent Oral Epidemiol 2015;43:2–8.

58. Davis R, Campbell R, Hildon Z, et al. Theories of behaviour and behaviour change across the social and behavioural sciences: a scoping review. Health Psychol Rev 2015;9:323–44.

59. Michie S, Richardson M, Johnston M, et al. The behaviour change taxonomy (v1) of 93 hierarchically clustered techniques: building an international consensus for the reporting of behaviour change interventions. Ann Behav Med 2013;46:81–95.

60. Cane J, O'Connor D, Michie S. Validation of the theoretical domains framework for use in behaviour change and implementation research. Implement Sci 2012;7:37.

61. Newlands R, Duncan EM, Prior M, et al. Barriers and facilitators of evidence-based management of patients with bacterial infections among general dental practitioners: a theory-informed interview study. Implement Sci 2016;11:11.

62. Schwendicke F, Foster Page LA, Smith LA, et al. To fill or not to fill: a qualitative cross-country study on dentists' decisions in managing non-cavitated proximal caries lesions. Implement Sci 2018;13:54.

63. Templeton AR, Young L, Bish A, et al. Patient-, organisation-, and system-level barriers and facilitators to preventative oral health care: a convergent mixed-methods study in primary dental care. Implement Sci 2016;11:5.

64. Gnich W, Bonetti D, Sherriff A, et al. Use of the theoretical domains framework to further understanding of what influences application of fluoride varnish to children's teeth: a national survey of general dental practitioners in Scotland. Community Dent Oral Epidemiol 2015;43:272–81.

65. Johnson MJ, May CR. Promoting professional behaviour change in healthcare: what interventions work, and why? A theory-led overview of systematic reviews. BMJ Open 2015;5:e008592.

66. Sbaraini A, Carter SM, Evans RW, et al. How do dentists and their teams incorporate evidence about preventative care? An empirical study. Community Dent Oral Epidemiol 2013;41:401–14.

67. Brocklehurst PR, Price J, Glenny AM, et al. The effect of different methods of remuneration on the behaviour of primary care dentists. Cochrane Database Syst Rev 2013;(11):CD009853.

68. Chandler J, Rycroft-Malone J, Hawkes C, et al. Application of simplified Complexity Theory concepts for healthcare social systems to explain the implementation of evidence into practice. J Adv Nurs 2016;72:461–80.

69. Damschroder L, Lowery JC. Evaluation of a large-scale weight management program using the consolidated framework for implementation research (CFIR). Implement Sci 2013;8:51.

70. Baker R, Camosso-Stefinovic J, Gillies C, et al. Tailored interventions to overcome identified barriers to change: effects on professional practice and health care outcomes. Cochrane Database Syst Rev 2010;(3):CD005470.

71. Baskerville NB, Liddy C, Hogg W. Systematic review and meta-analysis of practice facilitation within primary care settings. Ann Fam Med 2012;10(1):63–74.

72. McCormack B, Rycroft-Malone J, DeCorby K, et al. A realist review of interventions and strategies to promote evidence-informed healthcare: a focus on change agency. Implement Sci 2013;8(1):107.

73. Persson LA, Nga NT, Malqvist M, et al. Effect of facilitation of local maternal-and-newborn stakeholder groups on neonatal mortality: cluster-randomized controlled trial. PLoS Med 2013;10(5):e1001445.

74. Alla K, Hall WD, Whiteford HA, et al. How do we define the policy impact of public health research? A systematic review. Health Res Policy Syst 2017;15:84.

75. Eldridge SM, Lancaster GA, Campbell MJ, et al. Defining feasibility and pilot studies in preparation for randomised controlled trials: development of a conceptual framework. PLoS One 2016;11:e0150205.

76. Rycroft-Malone J, Seers K, Chandler J, et al. The role of evidence, context, and facilitation in an implementation trial: implications for the development of the PARIHS framework. Implement Sci 2013;8:28.

77. Murray E, Treweek S, Pope C, et al. Normalisation process theory: a framework for developing, evaluating and implementing complex interventions. BMC Med 2010;8:63.

78. Treweek S, Bevan S, Bower P, et al. Trial forge guidance 1: what is a study within a trial (SWAT)? Trials 2018;19:139.

79. Kirkham JJ, Gorst S, Altman DG, et al. Core outcome set–standards for reporting: The COS-STAR Statement. PLoS Med 2016;13(10):e1002148.

80. Listl S, Jürges H, Watt RG. Causal inference from observational data. Community Dent Oral Epidemiol 2016;44(5):409–15.

81. Colchero MA, Popkin Barry M, Rivera Juan A, et al. Beverage purchases from stores in Mexico under the excise tax on sugar sweetened beverages: observational study. BMJ 2016;352:h6704.

82. Wolpin KI. Ex ante policy evaluation, structural estimation, and model selection. Am Econ Rev 2007;97(2):48–52.

83. Bourguignon F, Spadaro A. Microsimulation as a tool for evaluating redistribution policies. J Econ Inequal 2006;4(1):77–106.

84. Anderson LM, Petticrew M, Rehfuess E, et al. Using logic models to capture complexity in systematic reviews. Res Synth Methods 2011;2(1):33–42.
85. Rohwer A, Pfadenhauer L, Burns J, et al. Logic models help make sense of complexity in systematic reviews and health technology assessments. J Clin Epidemiol 2017;83:37–47.
86. Goodwin T, Brocklehurst PR, Williams L, et al. How, and why, does capitation affect General Dental Practitioners' behaviour? A rapid realist review. Br J Healthc Management, in press.

Moving?

Make sure your subscription moves with you!

To notify us of your new address, find your **Clinics Account Number** (located on your mailing label above your name), and contact customer service at:

Email: journalscustomerservice-usa@elsevier.com

800-654-2452 (subscribers in the U.S. & Canada)
314-447-8871 (subscribers outside of the U.S. & Canada)

Fax number: 314-447-8029

Elsevier Health Sciences Division
Subscription Customer Service
3251 Riverport Lane
Maryland Heights, MO 63043

*To ensure uninterrupted delivery of your subscription, please notify us at least 4 weeks in advance of move.

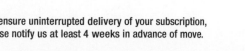
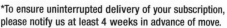

Printed and bound by CPI Group (UK) Ltd, Croydon, CR0 4YY

07/10/2024

01040501-0016